Fragments
Coping with Attention
Deficit Disorder

Fragments
Coping with Attention Deficit Disorder

Amy E. Stein, MSW

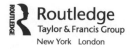

Routledge
Taylor & Francis Group
New York   London

First published by

The Haworth Press, Inc., 10 Alice Street, Binghamton, NY 13904-1580.

This edition published 2012 by Routledge

Routledge
Taylor & Francis Group
711 Third Avenue
New York, NY 10017

Routledge
Taylor & Francis Group
2 Park Square, Milton Park
Abingdon, Oxon OX14 4RN

PUBLISHER'S NOTE
Names of all patients, students, and clients of the MATE program discussed in this book have been changed to protect confidentiality.

Cover design by Jennifer M. Gaska.

Cover painting, "fragments," acrylic on canvas, © 1998 by Amy E. Stein.

Library of Congress Cataloging-in-Publication Data

Stein, Amy E.
    Fragments : coping with attention deficit disorder / Amy E. Stein.
        p. cm.
    Includes bibliographical references and index.
    ISBN 0-7890-1591-9 (hard : alk. paper)—ISBN 0-7890-1592-7 (soft : alk. paper)
    1. Attention-deficit disorder in adults—Treatment. 2. Attention-deficit hyperactivity disorder.
I. Title.

RC394.A85 S74 2002
616.85'89—dc21

                                                                            2002068936

for mom, dad, chris, and rebecca
with eternal love and gratitude

ABOUT THE AUTHOR

Amy E. Stein, MSW, earned her master's degree in social work from Rutgers University and graduated Cum Laude with a BA in psychology and a minor in professional writing. She has worked with adolescents for six years and implemented environmental education and art as alternative and experiential therapies. As a volunteer leader for five years at a Presbyterian church, she assisted in leading a program for middle and high school students, which included mission trips to refurbish and construct houses in Mexico and Maine. She has also worked as an addictions therapist in an inner-city hospital using a cognitive-behavioral model and counseled developmentally disabled adolescents in an alternative school where she implemented environmental education and art programs. Ms. Stein has been inducted into Psi Chi, the national honor society of psychology. She is also a member of the Pennsylvania Association for Sustainable Agriculture (PASA).

CONTENTS

Preface

This book is about life. It is written for those who think they have no hope, who struggle with life, decisions, addiction, and who search for themselves—any lost soul, really—but perhaps those who wander are not really lost, to paraphrase J. R. R. Tolkien. At the age of twenty-five, I was diagnosed with attention deficit hyperactivity disorder (ADHD), a "classic textbook case" in the words of the educational diagnostician. Although the criteria explained my impulsive and irrational behavior, it did not offer any pragmatic solutions other than medication and traditional psychotherapy, both of which failed me miserably. Medication served to merely mask my symptoms, and psychotherapy encouraged me to wallow in my problems. I discarded the Ritalin, as well as the diagnosis. Books and research on attention deficit disorder (ADD)/ADHD offered physiological explanations and also suggested medication and psychotherapy but again did not offer any true antidotes.

While skipping class one beautiful spring day during graduate school, I painted by a lake. Although the sky was brilliant blue filled with billowy masses of cumulus clouds, I smeared Mars black all over the surface of the canvas. I painted ultramarine blue spirals and haphazard black-and-white broken fragments of a mask until they disappeared into the center, trapped in a centrifugal force spiraling furiously downward. I have spent the past five years determined to break free from the suffocating clenches of this centrifugal force that pulls me into a downward spiral. Along this journey, many influential people have guided me and offered new directions, as are named in the acknowledgments and featured in the anecdotes within each chapter. I do not believe traditional psychotherapy or medication are solutions for those of us who fall under the label of ADD or ADHD.

Traditional psychotherapy, especially the Freudian school, tends to focus on the past. It is natural to desire explanations for behavior, but explanations take us only so far in life. We need to focus on *progression,* rather than regression, which consistently causes us to dredge up negative memories and allows the past to paralyze us. I refer to the proposed antidotes in this book as *progressive therapy*. Many people with ADHD tend to be highly creative and do not have anyone to nurture or encourage their creativity. Frustrated, they abandon any creative endeavors, repressing their emotions, which are then channeled into negative outlets, such as addiction.

This book is for those who suffer from the problems of ADD and ADHD. However, I do not fully believe in these labels. I believe that physiological differences distinguish those with ADD/ADHD from others, but these differences are more evident because of an educational system that promotes passive learning. The concept of experiential learning in schools today is, for the most part, confined to playgrounds at recess. As one solution, I propose that environmental education be incorporated into every educational curriculum. As further explored in Chapter 3, environmental education encompasses such subjects as math, English, history, science, social studies, art, and creative writing. It is hands-on, interactive teaching that is not confined within the four walls of a classroom, and it addresses the needs of students who *need* to be active.

Organic holism refers to a universe that is unified and interconnected, and our bodies are as such. Unfortunately, Western medicine tends to separate mind from body. We need a holistic approach for anyone who suffers from learning difficulties or depression. Oftentimes, depression accompanies the learning difficulties created from or exacerbated by our contemporary educational system. And, as I describe in greater detail in Chapter 1, I believe these learning difficulties and depression are evident only because the society that we live in bombards us with technology, encourages passive education that does not allow for movement, and promotes the disintegration of community. A holistic approach includes instilling a sense of community, nature, and spirituality; nurturing creativity; promoting exercise; educating people about the correlation between diet and behavior; and providing vocational direction with an emphasis on experiential careers and education.

Although the chapters in this book may initially appear to be mutually exclusive of each other, and at times the reader may wonder how they are possibly related to ADD/ADHD, the inherent relationship that exists between each chapter and the next comprises a holistic approach. For instance, how are the chapters on environmental education and religion related to each other? (And by the term religion, I do not refer to any one organized or unorganized religion. This can also be interpreted as spirituality.) Furthermore, how do these two factors simultaneously interact to affect those with ADD/ADHD, or anyone, for that matter?

Based on Scripture, God gave us this earth as a gift; we are merely tenants. This earth provides us with innumerable resources, such as land for growing food and lakes to quench our thirst, as well as homes for wildlife and vegetation, that are never to be taken for granted. Some of these precious resources are nonrenewable, meaning that if we do not practice conservation and preservation, we will rapidly deplete them simply through our ignorance. These resources relate to our well-being and affect our physical and emotional health. With ever-emerging technology, we are becoming a society that focuses on efficiency and productivity, which results in alienation from one another, ourselves, and the earth. Psychologically, we suffer as we consistently seek to fill a void in our lives, a fruitless search. We do not take the time to meditate, to hike in the forest and restore ourselves, to wade in streams, or to plant gardens. Socially, the concept of community disintegrates as reliance on technology as the sole entertainment increases. An emphasis on productivity and efficiency blatantly disregards the practice of sustainable living. We consume convenience foods laden with carcinogenic preservatives and do not take the time to grow our own vegetable gardens. Physically, our health suffers as a result of pesticide-sprayed crops produced by large-scale conventional farms that single-mindedly focus on profit at the expense of public health. Education assumes an assembly-line approach where overcrowded classrooms and weary teachers cannot address the needs of those who do not respond to the prescribed teaching curricula. These curricula do not take into consideration the needs of those who do not learn by the book. As with agribusiness, contemporary education is a centralized power that enslaves students and coerces them to pursue paths they do not choose.

The reader initially may not see any correlation between agriculture and ADD/ADHD. However, by enhancing one's diet, often a benefit of farming and gardening, health invariably improves. Chapter 4 describes essential fatty acids (EFAs) and the link between EFAs and ADD/ADHD. Furthermore, a study by a Princeton University professor discovered a correlation between movement and the brain neurotransmitter serotonin.[1] Those with ADD/ADHD often suffer from depression, which is linked with low levels of serotonin. Through constant movement, farming and gardening may boost serotonin levels. Farming, as a meditative activity, may induce alpha waves, another possible deficit in those with ADD/ADHD. Finally, these activities may lead to a sense of accomplishment, a new vocation or avocation, increased self-esteem, and enhanced self-efficacy. Margaret Mead (1934) postulated that a person's self-image depends in large part on his or her social image, as reflected in the eyes of others in his or her social group.[2] When people substitute a new society for their former one, their self-images are likely to change as well. The psychologist Albert Bandura proposed that self-efficacy is confidence in one's ability to conquer a task or challenge.[3] If one can learn to grow one's own food, is that not enhancing self-efficacy? Farming and gardening also build community, and through community, new relationships develop. I encourage you to explore these ideas further in Chapter 4.

Practicing sustainable living, praising the earth for its life-sustaining gifts, growing food or directly buying from farmers, and conserving water—these factors concurrently shape our behavior, our interactions with others, our educational system, and our health. Labels such as ADD/ADHD need not apply if we can relearn how to live *simply.* In our agrarian past, labels such as these did not exist because we *applied* concepts. Society consisted of active *and* interactive professions, such as farming, blacksmithing, and woodworking. Students were encouraged to pursue such occupations, and they certainly did not stay isolated indoors, vacant eyes staring at computer screens or televisions. Communities evolved and supported one another during times of hardship, thus instilling such values as loyalty, work ethics, and cooperation. Indian tribes, such as the Iroquois, practiced sustainable agriculture and lived in communally based extended families. Admirably, the Amish continue to build community and family relationships. Children and adults work together outside, maintaining their homesteads. I am not suggesting we live communally, but I ask that we carefully observe the values of other cultures and, in particular, their emphasis on community. Increasing technology breeds individuality and isolation, with society consistently placing a priority on productivity and efficiency. The concept of community, and its associated virtues, has disintegrated, resulting in an evolution of psychological disorders. Helen and Scott Nearing, authors of *Living the Good Life,* set a precedent by practicing and preaching a sustainable lifestyle through teaching others about the value of community and the preservation and conservation of natural resources.[4] Former urban professors disillusioned with the city, they abandoned their hectic lifestyles and fled to Vermont for solace and simple living. There, they planted abundant organic vegetable and fruit gardens, built a stone house, held weekly discussion groups about sustainable living, taught, wrote books, played music, and hosted thousands of transient people who were eager to adopt another lifestyle.

As alluded to earlier, I do not approve of labels, as they stigmatize and do not offer pragmatic solutions, but rather confinement in the traditional course of Western medical treatment. However, for the sake of simplicity, I will refer to ADD and ADHD as such throughout this book. Those diagnosed with ADD/ADHD simply have a different physiology, different cognitive wiring that the educational system does not understand. If we can implement change within the system, we may find that many ADD/ADHD symptoms are alleviated. It is time for progressive and experiential therapy, not regressive therapy that wallows in the past, allowing one to spend excessive time focusing on anger, depression, and negative thoughts. It is time for interactive and community experiences that build self-esteem, relationships, and new skills. Through sharing my personal experiences, I hope to incite interest in new vocations and avocations that will open doors for readers, especially those diagnosed with ADD/ADHD.

Acknowledgments

With love to Mom and Dad to whom I am eternally grateful for the gifts of independence, persistence, and art, for not giving up on me, and for not letting me give up on myself. I also thank Chris and Rebecca for the best sibling rivalry anyone could ever ask for; Tony for nine years; Reverend Craig Miller and Dr. Stewart Pattison for keeping me afloat, teaching me to swim, and answering all my questions. To my grandmothers, may your lights never extinguish. I thank my professor and mentor Kim Pearson for building a foundation for me; my professor Dr. Sally Archer for helping me in my pursuit of identity; Dr. Fred Rotgers and Carl Pfeifer for an open door and guidance; Professor Yvonne Johnson for an impromptu independent study that evolved into Chapter 3; Cake, Boobie, Anna Banana, and Nicky Noodle for sheltering and feeding me; Lisa, Michael, Sam, and Ben Katz for many wonderful meals and laughter; the "misfits" at the Coastal Learning Center for their priceless gifts (especially Cory); Scott Franzblau, a soulmate and wonderful teacher, as well as the first to enthusiastically read and edit "my fragments"; Jeff Hoagland and Rick Lear at the Stony Brook Millstone Watershed Association for their dedication and commitment to environmental education; the Murphys for loving me and being my other parents; Eileen, Paul, Ray, and MaryEllen for being my other siblings; Grace Wang for a door to always knock on and last-minute research help; Carolyn Sanchez for loving my paintings and keeping me at Rutgers; Anjali Khanna for getting me out of bed to class and graduation; David Gregory for helping me to evolve into a butterfly; Jeff Perlman for a midnight conversation on the dopamine D4 receptor gene; Cathy Haines for infinite words of wisdom; Lisa Bruschini and Dana McConnell for a summer at "the portsider" and eternal laughter; Lauren Ferreira, a kindred spirit; Candace Brennan for pedaling with me to the finish line; Eric Labacz for Rilke and conversations on art and solitude; Margaret O'Gorman and Mike Hunninghake for many inspirational forest conversations; Uncle Tim for starry, solipsistic nights; Uncle Mike; Judy (Dr. Judith Tingley), for giving me the right marketing tools; Marion, Karen, Shawn, Susan, and Jennifer for providing me with a hiatus and memorable West Coast adventures; Cousin Mick, for carrying my tricycle and me home; Aunt Effie and Uncle Minor for a lifetime dedicated to farming; Uncle Roy, Eric, Amy, Carly, and Chloe for encouraging me to keep painting; the cherished Tar Heels "street people" (especially Mrs. Schumann); John Mac-Farland for innumerable midnight conversations about life and callings; Tinicum Art and Science, especially John Heinz IV, for supporting all my endeavors; Buffy Morgan for "trying to change our brains and our lives" (and for many wonderful meals and art help!); Ellen Nenno for not kicking me out of English class and encouraging me to write; Roger Long for not kicking me out of art class and encouraging me to pursue art; my guidance counselor Patricia Coplin who insisted that I pursue my education; Andre Cantelmo and Hilary Niles for many memorable conversations at Heron Pond Farm; Evelyn Ramos for giving me the incentive to publish this; Jason Glick for slipping in some last minute research under my door; and Dutch Neck Presbyterian Church for my Christian roots. Much gratitude goes also to those who read and edited the manuscript during its growth; thank you for your wisdom: Scott Franzblau, Dr. Brian Donahue, Jeff Hoagland, Dr. Fred Rotgers, and editors Dr. Chris Merritt, Sharron Dorr, and Corrine Casanova for always encouraging me to take one more step; Dr. Robert Wildman for his belief in this book, Rebecca Browne at The Haworth Press for great assistance, Jennifer Gaska for her artistic skills, Peg Marr and Amy Rentner for their time and proficient editorial skills, and the writers who have profoundly influenced me: Henry David Thoreau, Vincent van Gogh, Brian Donahue, Wendell Berry, David Orr, Helen and Scott Nearing, Noel Perrin, and Theodore Roszak. Eternal thanks, love, and gratitude to everyone for believing in me long after I stopped believing in myself . . . this book would not be possible without the help and blessings of my wonderful family and friends.

cornfield

Lie in this barren field
sit amongst these seeds
implanted, rooting
burrowing deep into dark soil
Until rivets of water
trickle down
seeping into crevices
Stalks slowly emerge
pushing through the deep confines of this soil
upward
propelled toward the sky . . .
This field no longer barren
how simple to watch this surplus of growth
but yet wither inside . . .
So gather strength
walk away
and leave this field behind . . .

aes
3/26/96

Chapter 1

Piecing Together the Fragments

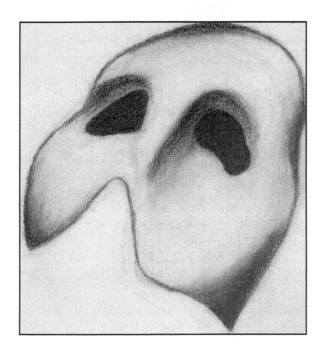

Life is like a game of cards.
The hand you are dealt is determinism;
the way you play it is free will.

Jawaharial Nehru

I walked up the long, winding driveway, listening to the sound of gravel crunch beneath my feet. A steady spring rain drizzled down my rain jacket and glistened on the canopy of green foliage. Majestic northern red oaks, shagbark hickories, and sugar maples lined the drive, and a bright green moss illuminated the forest floor. I gazed across the surrounding farm fields, the oats softly swaying in the fields adorned with hay bales. Stratus clouds converged in the distance, tinged with smudges of gray, appearing as if they had been randomly smeared across the sky with a wide, flat brush. I trekked past my favorite blue spruce and a row of Norway spruces, their lengthy cones dangling from the uppermost branches.

I am grateful to be walking in the cold, misty rain. I am grateful this journey leads me to my place of work. And I am grateful that I have ventured down many unknown paths to walk this one, although many past ones were ridden with unforeseen potholes and some with such an entangled thicket that I blindly groped my way along, led by faith alone. The thorns along the way sometimes tore at my flesh. My tears often blinded me, and I desperately wanted to collapse along the road, lie down in the nearby brush, and not emerge again. Ever. But someone always walked along and offered a hand, pulling me hesitantly along the way. God assumes many forms.

This particular driveway leads me to the site of an alternative school, a 137-acre farm in the mountains of eastern Pennsylvania. After years of stumbling down many a career path and fleeing from the confines of a classroom to other corners of the country and beyond, I found this haven of peace and freedom to teach, far from the constraints of traditional education, a place where one could learn and teach. We all assume both of these roles throughout our lives.

However, sometimes the ability to learn is precluded by the four walls of a classroom that do not permit one to venture beyond these boundaries. Like a plant deprived of essential light and water, one wilts and perhaps dies—not so much in the physical sense, but sometimes in the emotional sense, and perhaps this is worse. Contemporary society is often the root of the problem, failing to meet the needs of those who may march to the beat of a different drummer. Those who do are labeled as "behavioral" problems and their physiological deficits are disregarded. Pleas to pursue other cognitive paths of learning fall upon deaf ears. One can walk into a classroom these days and find many students slumped over their desks, defeated and helpless, lost without voices to express what they cannot yet understand. Fortunately, many of these lost souls are gifted in art, writing, and music, and these gifts become their salvation and outlet for raging emotions. However, they are often not nurtured because of the labels and diagnoses that are applied. Quick remedies are called for to mask the frustrations that manifest as behavioral problems as a result of learning disabilities. The student is labeled as having a learning disability, such as ADD, or a psychiatric disorder, but, for the most part, it is the institution with the learning disability.

Although this book focuses on ADD/ADHD and I refer to it as such throughout the book, this is the diagnosis that the medical profession applies to a particular set of physiological abnormalities. In turn, these "deficits" manifest as behavioral problems in the classroom because the majority of teachers present concepts in such a way that particular students cannot grasp. These "deficits" should not be referred to as such; rather, they should be referred to as "differences." Such physiological differences would not have been apparent in the past, as people were engaged in different jobs, many of which employed interactive and applied learning and skills. In the past, people with ADD would have excelled in trade professions. Those presently in careers such as investment banking and computer programming would have been at the mercy of farmers, woodworkers, blacksmiths, and others. It is my contention that so-called ADD/ADHD symptoms are apparent because education and occupations today drastically differ from those of the past. Fifty years ago, or even less, we would have been administering Ritalin or other stimulants and Prozac freely to everyone holding an office job, and *they* would have been the social outcasts. If students pursued these professions in schools or on farms of the past, they would have been put in detention for inactivity! As a result, accompanying emotional and psychological problems of ADD/ADHD inevitably surface leading to overdiagnosis and misdiagnosis of ADD/ADHD today. We are not seeking applicable solutions, but rather bandages in the form of Ritalin and other psychostimulant medication. If we increased our understanding of physiology, adjusted our teaching curricula, and stopped trying to encourage our students to pursue careers that guarantee high incomes, we might see a rapid decrease in the diagnosis of ADD/ADHD.

There are those who proclaim ADD/ADHD to be a hoax, but they have obviously not walked in the shoes of someone afflicted with the symptoms, which quickly become apparent as a result of our present educational system. A student diagnosed with ADD/ADHD faces being defeated, alienated, and stripped of any self-esteem by his or her experiences in the educational system, and it may take years to mend the damage done. Learning difficulties occur because students may be unable or unwilling to learn passively from a textbook, confined by the four walls of a classroom, or they may not want to pursue the particular career paths that society encourages today. Consequently, *this frustration evolves into depression, which in turn may result in relationship, career, and addiction problems, all so-called comorbid, or coexisting conditions of ADD/ADHD,* and it can cause a *lifetime* of damage. I still accept the physiological problems those with ADD/ADHD have, but I believe many of these physiological "deficits" would fade or diminish if our educational systems were different. Our teaching curricula do not meet the needs of those who possess a physiological brain structure that deviates from the norm. Studies of low levels of neurotransmitters indicate a role in depression, but, again, different teaching methods that incorporate active tasks, or experiential learning, may alleviate depression and mood swings. My objective in this book is to offer a repertoire of antidotes that may alleviate comorbid or coexisting disorders of ADD/ADHD; some or many of these may be incorporated into today's teaching curricula.

I do not endorse labels, as they serve to stigmatize, but for simplicity, I will refer to ADD/ADHD throughout this book. I will also deal with three specific subtypes of ADHD. The fourth revision of the *Diagnostic and Statistical Manual of Mental Disorders* (DSM-IV) lists three possible subtypes of ADHD: (1) ADHD, predominantly inattentive type, (2) ADHD, predominantly hyperactive-impulsive type, and (3) ADHD, combined type.[1] ADHD, predominantly inattentive type, is characterized by difficulty following through or sustaining attention, inability to listen to direction or focus on details in work or activities, often losing necessary materials, and being forgetful of daily activities. ADHD, predominantly hyperactive-impulsive type, is characterized by fidgeting, squirming, constant motion, excessive talking, interrupting, and difficulty waiting or taking turns. Combined type resembles a mixture of the previously described symptoms. Approximately 2 to 5 percent of school-aged children are diagnosed with ADHD.[2]

ADHD is one of the most common psychosocial disturbances observed in public schools, although most teachers are not educated or trained to provide the necessary accommodations. Children with ADHD experience low self-esteem, depression, and learning difficulties, resulting in lower academic achievement and risk of school failure. Furthermore, in one study, teachers revealed that their knowledge of ADHD did not come from research or formal education; 91 percent of respondents learned through their own experiences.[3] Because only a minority of children with ADHD are identified or receive health care interventions, the result is children with unmet mental health needs.

Students with ADHD have lower than expected or erratic grades and lower achievement and intelligence test scores caused by gaps in learned material, poor organizational and study skills, difficulty taking tests due to inattention and impulsivity, and failure to complete or turn in homework assignments. This population is at two to three times greater risk for school failure than their peers; over one-third do not complete high school, and 20 percent are at increased risk for substance abuse.[4] As many as 80 percent of diagnosed children continue to experience symptoms into adolescence, and up to 65 percent, into adulthood.[5]

Based on Section 504 of the Rehabilitation Act of 1973, accommodations are the first and primary method of providing support to students with a disability. The diagnosis of ADHD does not qualify a child for special educational services, but children with ADHD qualify under Section 504 for special assistance or appropriate learning accommodations. However, if the majority of teachers are not formally educated about ADHD, then critical interventions and accommodations cannot be implemented.

Social functioning is impaired as well, as peers quickly reject children with ADHD because of their aggression, impulsivity, and noncompliance with rules. Symptoms worsen when these students are placed in unstructured and minimally supervised, boring settings and circumstances that require sustained attention or mental effort. The majority of children with ADHD are placed in general education. Teachers within the general education classroom encounter significant challenges in managing the behavior of students with ADHD, yet one study revealed that "teachers' knowledge about consistent, effective classroom interventions seems to be limited" and "it appears that the interventions used with children who have ADHD are not consistent."[6] Furthermore, boys are four to nine times more likely to be diagnosed with ADHD, and children from low-socioeconomic-status families are less likely to see a primary care provider for emotional or behavioral problems.[7,8]

I have come quite a long way for someone who once refused to learn anything, almost failing ninth grade. Ever the acerbic child, I often quipped that I was "booked" if I received two detentions in one day. My assigned seat was in the front of the classroom, next to the teacher's desk. Exasperated teachers called to complain to my perplexed and frustrated parents. Lacking any organizational skills, I fell so far behind that it was useless even to study. I often perused the medicine cabinet, contemplating which pills would quickly end my misery. I spent many nights drawing intensely until the wee hours of dawn. It preserved my sanity.

During college, I worked thirty hours a week helping to manage an estate for a writer. I crammed for classes and pulled all-nighters because I could study for only thirty minutes at a time due to the innumerable distractions at home. I often feigned illness so as to make up tests. Although there were fewer distractions at school, I inevitably skipped half of my classes because I could not maintain an attention span for more than ninety minutes. My mind wandered so often I probably absorbed not more than fifteen minutes of any lecture. At the end of class, my notebook page would be blank and I would have to borrow friends' notes.

I did not lead a mundane existence as a child. My mother was convinced I had something doctors then referred to as "difficult child syndrome." She related stories of fighting with me when I was two concerning everything from clothing to bedtime. Apparently, I slept four hours and terrorized them for twenty. When I was older, my parents let me shower as long as I wanted because during that time I was not disruptive and creating pandemonium. They grimly referred to this as my "hydrotherapy." During adolescence, I left many a mark of fury on walls and doors. My parents retaliated by removing my bedroom door. Fortunately, my father retained his sense of humor and now jokes that he became quite adept at removing it from the hinges.

Little did I know that many distressing years would pass before I discovered the reasons for my behavior. One day in my late twenties during a summer internship on a nature preserve, we were wading into the lake, using a water ecology kit to test for pH, dissolved oxygen, and carbon dioxide. Water droplets splashed on my legs and the sun scattered a prism of scintillating lights on the invigorating water. The muddy bottom sand squished between my toes and tranquility enveloped me. Concepts clicked for the first time, and suddenly it made sense. I did not learn auditorily, passively in a classroom, or studying from a textbook. Any minute distraction led my attention elsewhere, and in the crowded, city high school I attended, this occurred every minute of the day. My minimal attention span combined with excessive energy meant I needed to learn visually, by doing. Engaged in hands-on, interactive activity, my mind did not wander and I made theoretical connections. Why did I not learn this way in the first place? Had visual and experiential learning been integrated into school, this may have saved me the interminable frustration and depression I battled throughout adolescence because of learning difficulties.

Roszak states that

> the time has come to move beyond the widely held belief that psychological health is solely a function of individual wholeness and nurturing human relationships. . . . This view exists within a framework that perpetuates the separation of person from world and that denies the essential importance of an individual's surroundings. . . . Our alienation from the rhythms of the natural world contribute, in a direct way, to our physical suffering.[9]

John B. Watson, the first behaviorist, argued vehemently that we should focus on directly, observable, measurable outward behavior. B. F. Skinner, one of the first psychologists to bring attention to resource depletion, pollution, and overpopulation, argued that we must redesign culture to shape more appropriate behavior.[10]

Furthermore, with the onslaught of managed care forcing therapists to cut service to clients, it is imperative that we recognize a need for alternative solutions. Recent experimental work has also shown that treatment must not be limited to the identified patient, his or her family, and the influence of peer systems. Community environmental factors must also be considered and integrated into treatment planning.

Kurt Lewin stressed the "eternal present," as it has been referred to in social psychology. Lewin believed that the key to understanding human social behavior lies in the present situation.[11] Frederick Perls founded Gestalt therapy, which focuses on holism: the sum of the parts is greater than the whole. Perls believed that in order to become conscious, one must examine the present, rather than irrelevant explanations from the past. Furthermore, Abraham Maslow, one of the founding fathers of humanistic psychology, argued that psychology focused on the negative, damaged, diseased parts of the human personality. As Maslow believed, the human being should strive to reach his or her full potential.[12]

Roszak sharply criticizes traditional psychology, especially its Freudian components. Modern psychotherapy is almost universally practiced during a fifty-minute hour in an office, in a building, in a city or suburb, completely alienating us from nature and disregarding our ecological unconscious. Steven Harper, an ecopsychologist, avoids using the word "therapy," which implies illness, a beginning and an end to treatment. He prefers to use the word "practice," which implies process, a lifetime of engagement and discovery, with no beginning or end.

Results of meta-analytic studies indicate that psychotherapy with delinquent adolescents results in little change following intervention, especially when the deviant behavior begins at an early age. However, cognitive-behavioral interventions that include social skills and problem-solving training have been successful. Delinquents will resort to ego defenses such as regression, and clinicians will be met with powerful resistance in the form of silence, pejorative remarks, and missed sessions. Without strong traditional values, adolescents may eventually turn to criminal behavior.

Although research and empirical studies document the necessity for alternative treatment, what is being done around the country? Advocacy and empirical studies are critical first steps, but implementation is an entirely different matter. Motivation, training, and education are mandatory for anyone working with adolescents. Environmental education is one solution to address the needs of those diagnosed with ADHD. Other experiential learning can involve integrating community service into schools, which will be presented in a later chapter. Incorporating even a few hours a week of any experiential learning may allow students to expend a certain amount of energy and thus would provide some focus for the time dedicated to traditional classes. I refer to this type of learning as *experiential* therapy, as well as *progressive* therapy. It provides knowledge that gives one the impetus to pursue a passion.

Learning difficulties and depression persisted throughout my adulthood. I dropped out of two graduate schools and resolved never to return. I ventured down various career paths, sometimes one a week, and worked as an editorial assistant, Internet writer, social worker, and freelance writer. Two weeks before my twenty-fifth birthday, my nine-year relationship with my boyfriend, Tony, mutually ended. We had spent little time together during the previous few years, both of us immersed in work and school. During our final argument, he stated, "You're a nonconformist with Peter Pan syndrome. You live for today, you don't think about tomorrow. Where are you going to be in five years, ten years? You have to start thinking about the future, and I can't live with someone who won't. You can't finish anything, you're too unfocused. You have too many dreams, you don't want to be tied to anything, not school, not a relationship. . . . You want to keep all your options open. I need someone stable, someone who won't decide to go run off and paint in the woods in five years" (I have).

Out of boredom and depression, one glass of wine always became another—and another—at any social gathering, beginning the first year of high school. The word "no" did not exist in my vocabulary. A few bottles of beer, a few glasses of wine, and a few mixed drinks clouded my senses and, for a night, I could live contentedly in a haze that far surpassed reality—except that it became reality. I often found myself waking up later on a cold lawn with no recollection of how I got there. I spent the next day nursing a headache and fatigue that diminished my energy and took precedence over a bike ride or a hike through the forest. I threw my precious time into a wastebasket, disposed of forever. I spent a lot of time in traffic court, battling speeding tickets and car accidents. Each time, I edged a little closer, teetering on the edge of a cliff and peering down onto the boulders. I wanted to fall sometimes, maybe for a moment to soar like an eagle. I felt trapped in a labyrinth, aimlessly wandering around, without any direction or knowledge as to what else existed other than a life inside the maze. I wanted to sever my past, to cut part of myself away like a sewing pattern and watch it fall to the floor in a shriveled pile.

I cherished and despised life. Some days I loved life with unrelenting passion—whether it was camping next to a crackling fire, mountain biking and inhaling the sweet lingering aroma of honeysuckle, kayaking down a sparkling river, writing a poem, painting by a lake, watching a sunset in Menemsha, thanking God I was alive to enjoy this beauty—but at the same time, I experienced a conflicting emotion of great sadness, knowing it was all temporary, at least on earth.

Who knows what awaits us after this life? And if such an afterlife exists, would you want to live forever in it?

I hated life at times because I wanted answers, but, then again, what could one ponder in life without the mystery? Mystery allows one to venture down interminable avenues of thought, exploration. What fun would life be if we had all the answers? No one would propose theories, discussions would be irrelevant, and we'd all be invested with the power of God. Other times, I hated life because I had no control over it. I didn't choose to come into this world, nor will I choose when to leave. At still other times, the brevity of life depressed me. The average life span is eighty years or so and, in the great scheme of things, that is a spit in the ocean. Someday all the people in my life will cease to exist and who will ever remember me, unless I manage to accomplish something significant enough to be etched indelibly into history books. The fleeting nature of life prompted me to question issues of faith and contemplate the concept of an afterlife.

I sought comfort in the Book of Ecclesiastes, written by a king of Israel referred to as "the philosopher." He concluded that existentialism was "useless and like trying to chase the wind." Bob Dylan concluded this as well in "Blowin' in the Wind." A Buddhist concept is to view the self as empty; a preoccupation with the search for oneself is fruitless. The writer of Ecclesiastes added:

> Whenever I tried to become wise and learn what goes on in the world, I realized that you could stay awake night and day and never be able to understand what God is doing. However hard you try, you will never find out. Wise men may claim to know, but they don't. (8:16-17)[13]

Furthermore, "if you wait until the wind and the weather are just right, you will never plant anything and never harvest anything." He concluded, "The best thing anyone can do is eat and drink and enjoy what he has worked for during the short life that God has given him; this is man's fate. No one remembers wise men and no one remembers fools; we all die, wise and foolish alike, the same fate awaits us all." In "Desolation Row," Dylan laments, "Her sin is her lifelessness."

Lifelessness afflicted me after spending one too many days cramped in a cubicle writing articles for an Internet Web site; ironically, it was a site for college students seeking career paths. Out of boredom and depression, I attempted graduate school again, this time in a Master's in Social Work program at Rutgers University. Yet another irony, my first-year graduate school internship was addictions counseling in an inner-city hospital at the Program for Addictions Consultation and Treatment (PACT), a unique program initiated by the Center for Alcohol Studies at Rutgers University, under the direction of psychologist Dr. Frederick Rotgers.

The internship was the only impetus that kept me in school. I could not maintain my attention for the three-hour classes, four required concurrently with an internship every semester for two years. I often left during the break, feeling a great sense of elation sweep over me, like an escaped prisoner. I managed to make a few 8:30 a.m. classes, but only a few. I was usually writing a paper into the wee hours of the morning, due that day. My good friend and next-door neighbor, Anjali, often called to drag me out of bed, without much success.

During my first semester at Rutgers, I stopped studying, eating, and sleeping. Restlessness plagued me every night. I paced around my room in the darkest and gloomiest of nights, staring out the frost-covered windows for hours, wishing I could silence all the thoughts in my head. I spent all semester diagnosing and assessing patients for major depressive episodes, and I sure as hell stepped into one myself, but I could not find a panacea for it.

One night, I sank into the bathtub and glanced at the smooth, creamy underside of my wrists and imagined slowly slicing open the skin with a single-edged razor, watching the blood trickle out and run down my arms in crimson streams, then branching out into tributaries. Was I using suicide as a way to test God? In a more rational light, we all make our choices. Suicide merely provided an escape from my feelings and emotions. It was the epitome of selfishness, and I could not leave my family to struggle with a lifetime of pain and unanswered questions. I needed to focus on my creative gifts, even as I squandered them.

Was I consistently sabotaging my own calling, simply always refusing out of fear to open my eyes to what lay before me? My friends were busy climbing corporate ladders and getting married, whereas I was still waiting by the side of the road or wandering aimlessly around the country, searching for something. I could not apply a label to myself: artist, writer, therapist? Was it lack of confidence in my work? Fear of commitment?

I regarded my creativity as a curse, not a gift. I focused on only what I didn't accomplish. People ponder over why van Gogh lopped off his ear. To me, there is no question. I wonder if his life would have been any different with the advent of therapy and antidepressants. Would his painting have suffered? Would he have rejected medication in favor of painting brilliant masterpieces? What if someone had taught him farming or gardening? He painted farmers, but from afar. Perhaps an intimacy with agricultural pursuits would have provided him the solace he needed.

Water and the forest often provided much solace for me and offered an escape from my overwhelming emotions, depression, and frustration. Martha's Vineyard is one favorite refuge where I found tranquility. I can never describe in words the overwhelming rush of inner tranquility and bliss that floods my body and mind when I am on this island. I leave behind all that is evil and bitter in the world. My family inexpensively rented an old Victorian on Church Street in Vineyard Haven for years and my cherished memories are of beating my brother at badminton in the spacious backyard, looking up from the outdoor shower at the beaming moon and starry night, and first venturing onto the nude beach in Gayhead when I was twelve. I remember standing in the clay pools in the cliffs, slathering red clay all over my body, then basking in the sun to dry and rinsing off in the chilly, but rejuvenating, New England waters.

I let my mind drift back to the flaming sunsets, hues of bright amber and maize on Menemsha Beach, watching the waves break against the cliffs overlooking West Chop, kayaking in the harbor, aimlessly wandering through outdoor art exhibits in Chilmark, swimming in the freshwater lake next to South Beach, created by an abundance of rain. Tony and I often rented bikes and logged miles and miles over the island, riding out to Long Beach through acres of forest and sandy trails, as well as to Chappaquidick to explore the Japanese gardens.

I wanted to create such a state of bliss wherever I was. I called Tony in tears one night. We still maintained a close friendship and he provided stability when I needed it.

"I give up. I don't know what to do anymore," I sobbed into the phone.

"What are you going to do, go to the island of misfit toys?"

I cried harder. "Do you know the little doll, who waits for Santa on Christmas Eve? My favorite line is the one where she cries, I haven't any dreams left to dream!"

Tony had a bootstrap philosophy. "Oh, come on. You have so much. Do you know how many people would trade places with you? Why don't you start focusing on something positive in your life?"

The tears suddenly ceased, and I felt extremely ungrateful for what God had given me. In desperation, I made a beeline for the student health center and talked to a very kind physician, who referred me to an educational diagnostician on campus. After a lengthy interview and giving me forms for doctors and my parents to complete, she diagnosed me with ADHD at age twenty-five. I read everything I could on ADHD but still denied that it existed. I was referred to a psychiatrist (who I believe had ADHD herself) who wanted to argue that I did not have ADHD. I did not return after the first session and found a doctor who specialized in ADHD. He prescribed sixty milligrams of Ritalin daily, and I spent twelve to fifteen hours per day in a drug-induced slumber. I felt like a deer, frozen in the glare of oncoming headlights. I feared I would wind up a homeless vagabond, curled up on a park bench, clutching on to a scrap of blanket for dear life. A rolling stone, in the immortal words of Bob Dylan. No direction home. I wanted to drift from job to job and constantly change my environment, but through her clenched teeth my mother said, "That's how people become homeless!"

I quickly discarded the Ritalin and packed my belongings, registered for a leave of absence at Rutgers, and hopped on a plane bound to Chicago to visit my brother with my meager life savings. I am a descendant of a long line of vagabonds, lost souls, artists, and writers. My relatives have wandered through life, fleeing to the West Coast, seeking refuge with relatives in times of turbulence. I suddenly wanted to swim, not sink. I was tired of treading water, barely holding my head up. I sought a new life, a new beginning. The Latin phrase "tabula rasa" is appropriate. But first, I just needed to "be" for a while.

Chicago

The rain drizzles steadily outside and I watch mesmerized, as it trickles down the dusty windowpanes. My brother, Chris, the youth director at a church in a suburb of Illinois, is in a meeting, and I assume it will be a while. I swivel around in the chair and something catches the corner of my eye. It is a simple pen-and-ink drawing of a lighthouse situated on an island. I shuffle through some papers until I find a blank sheet, then rifle through a drawer for a pencil. I pick up the pencil and caress the smooth wooden grooves between my thumb and forefinger and start to sketch the outline of the lighthouse. Suddenly, like magic, overwhelming feelings of familiarity flood me and I have traveled back to my early teenage years when I drew into the early hours of the morning, forcing myself to succumb to slumber. For the next hour, I immerse myself in the drawing, escaping into the dissociative state of mind I enter once I begin drawing, oblivious to the passage of time. So engrossed in the drawing, I fail to hear Chris walk into the room and tap me on the shoulder; the effect is similar to a hypnotist snapping his client out of a trance. I jump and drop the pencil on the desk. He looks over my shoulder as I hurriedly fold the paper.

"Are you finished yet?" I ask, feigning annoyance, although I feel nothing but an inner sense of tranquility.

"Yup. You ready?"

"Been ready."

"What are you drawing?" he asks.

"Nothing, just messing around."

We walk out into the parking lot. I've already been here four days, simply relaxing, reading, essentially doing nothing but observing others living their lives. I have plans to leave tomorrow to stay with my cousin Karen for a while, but I do not make any definite plans as to what I will do once I am there, or how long I will stay.

Arizona

My cousin Karen is finishing her undergraduate degree and is in the midst of a flurry of papers. She is kind enough to supply me with extra tickets to baseball spring training my first week and to take me to Arizona State University to wander around the campus. One weekend, Karen, her boyfriend, Shawn, and I fly to San Diego for the day, and it costs $20 round trip, thanks to her discount as a flight attendant. In San Diego, we rent a fire engine red convertible and cruise up to Mission Beach. It is a beautiful day, and we wander around the beach, watching the seals basking in the sun. How nice to be one of those seals, a life devoid of responsibility, bills, agendas. I suppose I am living that life right now, albeit temporary. We spend the remainder of the day driving along the Pacific, hopping out onto beaches, and finish the day sipping cappuccino on a restaurant deck, watching the sunset's streaks of lilac fade into yellow.

I spend three weeks in Arizona, divided between my cousin's house and my uncle's house. I had spent some time in Arizona five years ago and explored the Grand Canyon and breathtaking Sedona. However, I really have no desire to sightsee this time and spend the days aimlessly wandering into museums, jogging during sunset, and reading sporadically. I do not paint; I do not write. I do spend some time hiking Squaw Peak and South Mountain with my aunt and uncle on weekends, and I am happy finally to climb a literal mountain, instead of a metaphorical one. My uncle's wife, Judith Tingley, is a psychologist, and I am fascinated with her collection of books, including the ones she has written. In a lawn chair under a grapefruit tree I read a book about healing from long-term relationships. The author, Bruce Fisher, discusses the roles of the dumper and the dumpee and compares the demise of a relationship to Elisabeth Kübler-Ross's stages of death and dying. I had already advanced through every stage: denial, anger, bargaining, grief, and acceptance. However, I find myself sometimes repeating stages, or regressing once I think I've reached acceptance. I assume it is a circular process, one that can be repeated many times and that varies from individual to individual.

On St. Patrick's Day, Karen, Shawn, and I go to a bar in Tempe to see a blues band. After a couple of hours, we decide to leave, but on the way out, I spot a woman hunched over a table in the corner reading cards. A scarf swathes her head and cascades over her shoulders. I tap Karen on the shoulder, and we venture over.

The woman is dealing tarot cards and speaking to someone.

"Should I do it?" I ask Karen.

"Yeah, why not? It'd be interesting."

I wait impatiently. Since childhood, the sixth sense has always intrigued me. I voraciously read many books on telepathy, clairvoyance, and telekinetic energy. Innumerable supernatural stories about my grandparents' house in northern Massachusetts have fascinated my family for decades. Finally, she is finished and I anxiously sit down. She explains the chakras and how energy called ch'i moves through the body. She asks if she may pray before reading the tarot cards. I am surprised but agree without hesitation. She asks for guidance during the reading and then doles out the cards on the table.

"You're very anxious and worried and you don't need to be," she begins. "You're very family-oriented, have high values." I don't say anything but merely nod and try to maintain a poker face. She peers over her glasses.

"You feel like you're out in the cold, you're traveling, searching . . . no job and no money." She places another card on the table. "You feel as if you're blindfolded, stumbling . . . trying to break away from old patterns, establish new ones." So far she is speaking in generalizations that could apply to many people my age. On the other hand, I could be working full-time and be perfectly satisfied with my life. I ask what direction my career path will take. "Something is being offered to you and you are refusing to accept it or ignoring it. You won't do what you studied in school." I had no intention of pursuing psychology. I ask about relationships, specifically Tony. "You'll stay in contact and remain friends." What I expected to hear. I ask about any future relationships. "He has a woman in his life, married or something, but she will terminate the relationship. Oh! This next card is the most powerful one in the deck. God is guiding this relationship." She looks up at me. "Don't hurry it," she says knowingly. "Don't hurry it." Hurry what? I cannot imagine ever maintaining another relationship, let alone trying to hurry one. She cleans up the cards and a man hovers over me, also anxious for his turn. If psychics or sages can predict the future and such an event does later occur in an individual's life, would that not support the concept of some predetermined destiny? Does God intervene in our lives, sometimes by speaking through others? Do we truly have free will to make our own choices or do we follow a calling that we hear, one that is chosen for us? Life holds so many mysteries to unravel.

California

Flying stand-by has its advantages; I can leave when I want. Early one morning, I wake once again to bright sunshine streaming into my room. Northern California beckons. I miss spring, waking up to cloudy mornings, and the ominous skies warning of an impending thunderstorm.

I bid farewell to Karen and profusely thank her, then fly to San Francisco to seek refuge with my other cousin Jennifer. Northern California appeals to me, more reminiscent of the East Coast with cloudy days and a splendor of green fields meeting the horizon. The next few days, I wander around San Francisco alone and contentedly stroll along Fisherman's Wharf, sample chocolate at Ghiradelli Square, and stay with a friend in Nob Hill. For any artist, writer, or musician, solitude is conducive as well as critical for the creative process. One needs to delve into the inner depths of the mind and that requires much solitude and peace without distraction. Compromise is not necessary when one is alone. Solitude also allows exploration and wandering into unchartered territories without the distraction of a companion.

One morning, I ride a cable car down to the wharf to find a bike shop. I rent a mountain bike and ride to the Golden Gate Bridge. At the base, I pause and stare at the massive conglomeration of wires and steel supporting tons of weight, appearing suspended in midair. I take a deep breath and begin the journey across the bay. The wind whips through my hair and the brilliant sunshine beams down upon me. Exhilarated, I stop midway to observe the city, now a small collection of buildings in the distance. I begin the descent of the latter half and cycle into Marin County, touring Sausalito for a while. It is a little town crowded with art galleries and cafés on the water. I lock my bike in a rack and wander into an art gallery. A middle-aged man hunches over a canvas in a back room, and the distinct odor of turpentine is familiar.

"Are you looking for anything in particular?" he asks, looking up at me, seeming slightly distracted.

"No, just browsing. How long have you been painting?"

"Well, most of my life. My wife is an artist, also." He motions to some watercolor paintings of various flowers on the wall. "We've had this studio for twenty-seven years." His face brightens, and he eagerly walks over to show me his paintings displayed on the walls.

"I used to do a lot of still life, but now I'm doing a lot of abstract still life."

"Yeah, I was always into abstract stuff," I say, nodding.

"You paint?"

"I drew throughout elementary school, middle school, and high school. I'd stay up all night drawing and only go to bed when my parents forced me to." I wistfully laugh at the memory. "I painted a lot in my high school art class. I miss it."

"So why don't you start again?"

"I don't know why I stopped. Got involved in a relationship, everything else went down the tubes, including my identity. I think it's only fear now." I smirk. "Hmph. Only."

"The hardest thing to do is not to paint. The painter Willem de Kooning once said, 'It's absurd to pursue art, but it's absurd not to.' "

"It is. Art is my form of expression and I've denied myself that expression for many years.... So, how do I start getting my stuff out?"

"Build up a portfolio and promote yourself. Being an artist is ninety percent promotion, and it's the only way you'll get anywhere. Call your local arts council; send slides to them and maybe you'll get an exhibit. Coffeehouses also exhibit local artists. It's getting started that's the most difficult part. Once you get beyond that, it often snowballs."

"You seem really happy."

"Like I said, I've been here twenty-seven years." He pauses and stares off into space. "You need to get bitten," he says, clenching his fist for emphasis. "To be an artist, you can't think about anything else; you can't divide yourself." He swabs his brush around on the palette. I thank him and walk outside, glancing at my watch. Just enough time to catch the ferry and return my bike.

I share my day with Jennifer who is working at home to build a business. We make plans to camp in Yosemite for the weekend, pack, and leave the next morning. The two-hour drive east of San Francisco takes us up narrow, winding mountain roads. From my passenger window, the disappearing roads appear to be long stretches of gray ribbon winding through a dense foliage of leaves. Once we enter the park, patches of snow still dot the landscape. We stop along the way to snap pictures of the valley below, great gorges carved from glaciers, reminiscent of miniature Grand Canyons. The Merced River winds its way past Half Dome, a rock mass cut in two by erosion, situated 4,730 feet over Mirror Lake. The surrounding mountain hemlock, fir, sugar pines, maple, oak, and Pacific dogwood trees reflect an array of beautiful shapes and shadows in the water. I plan to paint this captivating scene by referring to photographs. Massive granite formations surround Bridalveil Falls, a cascading veil of water falling 620 feet over Cathedral Rocks, and a fine mist falls another 300 feet into Bridalveil Creek. Bridalveil Falls was formed from glacial ice. Yosemite Falls plunges 2,425 feet from Yosemite Creek; it is the tallest waterfall in North America. The Mariposa Grove, a splendor of sequoias, boasts over 500 mature trees, including the Grizzly Giant, standing 209 feet at 2,700 years old. We park along the road and hike past El Capitan, a 3,600-foot-high granite monolith, and watch what we assume to be rock climbers strategically ascend the mass. From a distance, our eyes can discern only moving specks.

It is early evening by the time we set up a campsite, surrounded by the stately sequoias. We build a fire and Jennifer unpacks a cake for my twenty-sixth birthday. Her husband and a friend are with us, and they harmoniously sing a birthday song. After we enjoy some California wine from a Napa Valley vineyard, I sleep peacefully in my tent until I awake in the middle of the night to rumbling thunder, then drift back to sleep to the rhythm of a steady rain. Unfortunately, it is only an overnight trip, and we have to leave the next morning after a brief hike. Once we return to Jennifer's, restlessness strikes and I fly home the following week.

* * *

Is restlessness so awful? I find that it is a common characteristic in those diagnosed with ADD/ADHD. These restless souls often include artists who paint beautiful mountains from their travels, musicians who sing of those other restless souls they meet along their travels, and writers whose prose describes their journeys, enticing readers to embark on similar expeditions. However, many environmentalists condemn restlessness, insisting that planting roots is crucial for the well-being of the planet and for building community relationships. In *Ecological Literacy,* David Orr posed the question: Are immobility and rootedness synonymous? My answer is an affirmative no, although they are not mutually exclusive of each other. I believe one can be rooted, yet still mobile. Friends and family have taught me to plant roots, literally and figuratively. I have planted abundant gardens, established relationships with neighbors, and worked and written for several environmental organizations. Yet, I still crave excitement and adventure, biking, hiking and kayaking in New England, where I spent many happy childhood days, finding refuge and healing in nature.

Psychologist Frederick Perls believed that unconsciousness results from a fragmentation of various parts of the psyche; awareness brings about an integration of these dissociated parts.[14] A similar dissociative split often occurs between spirit and nature. If we do not experience our own body, instincts, and sensations, this separation projects outward, and we perceive ourselves as separate from the earth.

In his book *The Unsettling of America,* Wendell Berry describes fragmentation as a disease, a disconnection of the body from the soul.[15] Berry states that the societal response is a self-indulgent identity crisis and that the cure is autonomy. In defense, not all people are fortunate enough to stumble upon a path in life they want to travel and pursuing a calling requires abundant time and much self-reflection. During my travels, I was not seeking autonomy; I was seeking explanations and a way to integrate the fragmentation I experienced. Perhaps I have been unconscious most of my life; it took that long to decipher my erratic behavior and discover the cure for my ailments. Travel may be a preparation for a calling later in life.

My travels satisfied my wanderlust and inspired me. Without them, I would have stagnated; many of my paintings and writings would not exist. These travels helped to define my identity . . . the people I met along the way have enhanced and irrevocably changed my life, guiding me in new directions. Part of the journey of life is to discover exciting facets of one's personality. Certainty is boring. What a mundane existence if one knew everything about oneself from the time of birth!

What accounts for the depression, addiction, and learning disabilities with which many people with ADD/ADHD battle? There are several physiological theories: low levels of dopamine, reduced blood flow in the frontal lobes of the brain, and a disturbance in the reticular activating system. Dopamine is a neurotransmitter in the brain that has been shown to play a role in depression. The frontal lobes of the brain are responsible for emotion, planning, and initiative, common problems faced by people with ADD/ADHD. Frontal lobe brain damage causes impulsivity, mood swings, and hyperactivity, all symptoms of ADHD. Three brain regions control attention and behavior: the prefrontal cortex, part of the basal ganglia, and the vermis region of the cerebellum. These regions are significantly smaller in children with ADHD.[16]

The reticular activating system (RAS) is a finger-shaped network of neurons, extending from the spinal cord to the thalamus, located in the brain stem. Sensory input travels up the spinal cord to the thalamus, where some of it branches off and activates the RAS, which filters incoming stimuli, blocking out irrelevant noises. Someone with ADHD may complain of sensitivity to noise or a feeling of being bombarded with extraneous stimuli. The RAS failing to filter stimuli properly provides the basis for this feeling. It is analogous to receiving all the signals for one radio station. The RAS and the frontal lobe interact as a communication feedback loop, and some researchers have postulated that there is a malfunction within this loop.[17] The RAS is also the arousal system, regulating the state of alertness from deep sleep to full, waking consciousness. That many people with ADHD struggle to stay alert and pay attention suggests impairment in this system. Although it often takes hours for me to feel fully awake, I find that when I sleep consistently (i.e., go to bed and rise at the same hours every day), exercise, and take vitamins, this problem is greatly alleviated.

The National Institute of Alcohol Abuse and Alcoholism (NIAAA) cites studies that low-serotonin individuals often develop hypoglycemia (low blood sugar). Hypoglycemia is common in people with ADHD. Deficiencies in serotonin increase irritability and aggression, impulsivity, violent suicide, alcohol and drug use, eating and bingeing, sexual activity, insomnia, and disruption of circadian body rhythms.[18] Perhaps this accounts for those individuals who feel they lack a "physiological off switch."

A study of rhesus monkeys (greater than 90 percent DNA sharing) indicated that those with the lowest levels of serotonin exhibited the most violent behavior.[19] Monkeys with higher serotonin activity took the trouble to move branch to branch to shorten leaping distances. Those with lower serotonin impulsively leaped great distances at heights where falls could prove fatal. This offers one explanation for the impulsive behavior exhibited by those with ADHD. Studies show that drugs which increase serotonin activity reduce aggression, while those which decrease serotonin activity heighten aggression. Serotonin restricts neural information and inhibits the intensity of signals; decreased serotonin function results in an overload of signals, and this may produce erratic behavior, such as hyperactivity.

Throughout my research, I noticed that people with addiction problems had decreased P300 waves, and other studies cited learning and memory problems—all problems that those with ADD/ADHD may encounter. Brain waves are measured in hertz, units of frequency equivalent to one cycle per second. Beta waves (13-30 Hz) are usually associated with wide-awake, alert, problem-solving modes of thought. Theta (5-7 Hz) waves are related to dreaming or creative activities. Delta waves (.5-4 Hz) are associated with dreamless sleep. Alpha waves (8-12 Hz) correspond to relaxation and contemplative, meditative states.[20] P300 denotes a wave of brain electrical activity emerging approximately 300 milliseconds (ms) after the presentation of a rare or surprising stimulus, especially when the occurrence of the stimulus must be actively acknowledged by the subject (i.e., pressing a response key).[21] The "P" stands for a positive voltage potential and 300 represents a 300 ms poststimulus brain reaction. Its amplitude increases with unpredictable, unlikely, or highly significant stimuli and is therefore considered a measure of mental activity. Amplitude refers to the height of brain waves that determine loudness; a greater amplitude increases sound. P300 waves in the brain have been associated with addiction, attention, workload, stimulus classification, response selection, expectancy, surprise, extraction of information, transfer of information into consciousness, memory, and learning. [22, 23]

MRIs suggest that P300 waves recorded from the scalp originate from neural generators in the frontal and parietotemporal regions of the brain, tend to be frontally distributed, and are disrupted by lesions of the dorsolateral frontal cortex.[24, 25, 26] Considering that one of the physiological theories of ADD is reduced blood flow in the frontal lobes of the brain, and hence affects emotion, planning, and thinking, this may provide evidence for a correlation between a disruption of P300 waves in people with ADD and the subsequent physiological effects. Methylphenidate (Ritalin) has been found to increase P300 waves by 30 percent in those diagnosed with ADD/ADHD.[27]

Studies with adolescents with conduct disorder problems and ADD/ADHD have found persistent responses in P300 waves pertaining to specific tasks and decreased P300 amplitudes in different locations of the brain at specific ages. In a study of adolescents diagnosed with conduct disorder, adolescents with more conduct disorder problems exhibited *smaller* P300 amplitudes than subjects without any conduct disorder problems. However, this study was age specific. Adolescents under the age of 16.5 years had lower P300 amplitudes within the posterior region of the brain. Among adolescents older than 16.5 years, the effects of conduct problems had shifted toward the *frontal* region of the brain. This may be attributed to delayed brain maturation and is deduced from the high amount of slow wave and low amount of alpha wave typical in the normal, but immature EEGs of healthy, younger children.[28] The frontal lobe is the last area of the brain to mature, and it regulates higher-level cognitive operations, including foresight and impulse control—all difficulties faced by those with ADD/ADHD. Furthermore, P300 decrements persist into adulthood and may be present in those with adult antisocial personality disorder and/or other adult psychiatric disorders, including substance abuse.[29] In addition, quantitative EEG measures have differentiated between the specific subtypes of ADD, as well as more delta, fast theta waves and fewer alpha waves in children with ADHD, which again suggests a delay in the maturation of cerebral inhibitory function.[30,31]

One possible approach to dealing with brain wave disruption is relaxation exercise. Meditation can induce alpha brain waves that are associated with relaxation.[32] Thus, perhaps other meditative activities mentioned in this book, such as writing, painting, farming, and hiking, may also induce alpha waves, eliminating ADD/ADHD comorbid disorders. People often scoff that those with ADD/ADHD could ever meditate. It seems paradoxical, but it is possible with perseverance and should indisputably be included as one panacea for ADD/ADHD, thus its inclusion as a separate chapter. From my personal meditative experiences, dissociative states of mind can enhance meditation. Not everyone has the ability to achieve a dissociative state, and I believe those with ADD/ADHD have more of an inclination to dissociate, a trait often found among musicians, artists, and writers, many of whom are diagnosed with ADD/ADHD.

Other studies measured P300 waves during passive and active tasks, and this may be generalized to passive classroom learning compared to active or experiential learning. Passive tasks do not elicit P300 waves identical to those elicited during active tasks; P300 components decreased in amplitude during passive tasks.[33] Even more interesting, P300 waves decreased with *repeated passive* tasks, especially for *auditory* stimuli, fostering a resistance to habituation. One might infer that this could be generalized to a classroom lecture format and would explain the difficulty that students with ADD/ADHD have in sustaining their attention in such an environment.

In another study of eleven sixteen-year-old males and females, free from medication affecting brain activity, a significant decrease in evoked auditory (i.e., a low- or high-pitch tone) P300 amplitude was discovered when participants were asked to perform both auditory and visual tasks simultaneously.[34] Thus, this might be evidence that people with ADD/ADHD work better on one task at a time as opposed to multiple tasks. I have witnessed many a student abandon a task if he or she initially views it as comprised of simultaneous tasks that appear overwhelming. Thus, if the overall task is broken down into a sequence of *single* tasks, the student will be able to work steadily and confidently toward a tangible goal. When a subject performs a task requiring sustained attention, novel stimuli that are irrelevant or a secondary task often elicits a P300 component. Thus, this may explain why people with ADD become so easily distracted. Another type of distraction occurs when students are bombarded with external stimuli. Distracting subjects by requiring them to pay attention to stimuli from several modalities reliably reduces P300 amplitude.[35] As a result, students tend to experience confusion over which task to attend to first and begin to feel overwhelmed.

In addition, a persistent P300, short-latency wave (330-470 ms) throughout an auditory task has been found in easily distractible children, whereas nondistractible children experience a decrease in wave size toward the end of the task. Typically, short-latency, frontally distributed P300 responses are elicited by only *novel* or surprising stimuli. Nonnovel auditory target stimuli may activate the brain's orienting networks in easily distractible children.[36] For instance, if I try to read a journal article in the library, I must isolate myself in a corner desk. Otherwise, I am distracted by *every* conversation and noise, and I lose all concentration. This means that I must repeatedly read everything or I absorb little of the content. Improved resistance to distraction characterizes normal development; those with ADD/ADHD experience increased distractibility. In the classroom, this is often perceived as a behavioral problem instead of a deficit in the brain's ability to process information. P300 waves normally decrease in size when stimuli lose their novelty through repetition. Persistent activity of P300 waves in the right frontal lobe suggests that distractible children continue to show enhanced orientation to stimuli that should have been encoded or categorized.

As addiction may be a comorbid symptom in those with ADD/ADHD, it is not surprising that abnormalities in P300 waves recorded from substance-dependent patients do not disappear even after long periods of abstinence. P300 amplitude decrements are still detectable in alcohol-dependent patients after one year of abstinence. In cocaine-dependent patients, P300 amplitude decrements, particularly over the frontal areas of the brain, are equally persistent. However, these P300 decrements have been found to exist *prior* to the onset of substance abuse. Studies of the biological offspring of alcohol-dependent fathers demonstrated P300 decrements similar to those found in their alcohol and drug-dependent parents, perhaps indicative of a genetic component. It is still unknown whether this is a coincidence or a direct etiologic contribution to risk for substance dependence. However, P300 decrements are repeatedly demonstrated among individuals with no family history of substance dependence.[37]

P300 waves may be increased through yoga (see Chapter 7) and taking omega-3 supplements (see Chapter 4). One study discovered that P300 waves increased when healthy adults were given docosahexaenoic acid (DHA), an omega-3 fatty acid, which improved mental abilities such as memory and learning. This rate decreases with age and is noticeably slower in people with dementia.[38] What exactly is the relationship between P300 waves and omega-3 fatty acids? Is it limited to DHA? How does this impact ADD/ADHD? I may only hope that this prompts researchers interested in ADD/ADHD to investigate this line of questioning further in empirical studies.

Sudarshana Kriya Yoga (SKY), when practiced as a sole treatment for thirty minutes daily for three months, increased P300 amplitude and also improved symptoms of dysthymia, normalizing at three months.[39] Those with ADD/ADHD may suffer from dysthymia. According to the DSM-IV, dysthymia is a depressed mood for the majority of the day for a period of at least two years for adults and duration of one year for children and adolescents. Symptoms include poor appetite or overeating, insomnia or hypersomnia, low energy or fatigue, low self-esteem, poor concentration or difficulty making decisions, and feelings of hopelessness.

Although much skepticism exists regarding ADD/ADHD and over-diagnosis is rampant, studies provide evidence of a genetic and physiological basis. Investigations of brain studies and function using magnetic resonance imaging (MRI), positron-emission computed tomography (PET), and photon-emission computed tomography (SPECT) have shown significant differences between healthy controls and subjects with ADHD and more than twenty family or genetic studies implicate the role of genetic factors.[40] Another study concluded there is a "substantial genetic component."[41]

Furthermore, empirical studies were conducted that show a genetic relationship between ADHD and a specific genetic polymorphism residing within the dopamine D4 receptor gene (DRD4). Polymorphisms are changes in the DNA sequence of a particular gene between two individuals. These polymorphisms can be detected by DNA sequence analysis and arise as single base substitutions, deletions or insertions, or as multiple repetitions of a particular sequence of base pairs (bp). If a particular polymorphism is repeated from generation to generation and if a correlation exists between individuals with this polymorphism and the incidence of a particular disease, then scientists have evidence that either that gene or an adjacent gene contributes to the disease. Interestingly, polymorphisms have been detected in the DRD4 gene; a 1996 study discovered an association between novelty-seeking behavior and the DRD4 gene. Researchers were interested in polymorphism that exists as an expansion of a repetitive sequence within the gene, called the 7-repeat allele. As novelty-seeking behavior is common in those with ADHD, this finding led to a study on ADHD and the DRD4 gene. Scientists discovered an increased frequency of the 7-repeat allele (the form of a gene) in those children diagnosed with ADHD-inattentive subtype. A genetic study of siblings also replicated these findings; the sibling with the greater 7-repeat alleles displayed more inattentive symptoms than the cosibling with fewer 7-repeat alleles. These expanded repeats in the DRD4 gene may increase the susceptibility to ADHD.[42]

This gene mutation results in an altered receptor and a possible decreased sensitivity to dopamine. Dopamine is released at the presynaptic terminal, diffuses across the synaptic cleft, and binds to specific dopamine receptors on the membrane of the postsynaptic terminal. The body may produce a normal amount of dopamine, but the neurons cannot bind it as well and this in turn affects behavior.[43]

Matthew, a fifteen-year-old student at the alternative school where I spent my second-year internship, rocked back and forth on the legs of his chair. He opened and closed all the desk drawers, rooting through papers. He paused and squinted at me from across the desk in my office. A restless soul, he could not stay in a classroom for more than fifteen minutes. Matthew's poor teacher spent most of her day trying to track him down. At fifteen, he often came to school high on marijuana and recounted tales of acid trips and binge drinking. Acting on impulse one day, he decided to take his father's car for a spin. His final destination turned out to be a jail cell and mandatory thirty-day inpatient rehabilitation. They handed Matthew to me.

I worked with Matthew most of the school year. One day he said to me, "You're one of two people that doesn't make me feel like a piece of shit." I attempted to explain ADHD.

"What do you do when you go to a swimming pool?" I inquired.

"Jump in," he said, shrugging without hesitation.

"Exactly. People with ADHD jump in without testing the water first. But sometimes this works out. It's the people with ADHD who take chances and initiate great inventions or organizations. Other times, the water may be scalding or freezing and the result is hypothermia or a burn. People who test the water may stick their toes in, but they withdraw them if the temperature is not right."

Matthew folded his arms assuredly and sat back in his chair. He stated, matter-of-factly, "Miss, I don't think you test the waters." He caught me off guard. I hesitated before speaking and carefully chose my words.

"Well, Matthew . . . I've learned to test the waters after a lot of life experience. But I've been frozen and I've been burned."

Dr. Daniel Amen, author of *Change Your Brain, Change Your Life,* believes that ADD occurs as a result of neurological dysfunction in the prefrontal cortex of the brain. The prefrontal cortex is the front third of the brain underneath the forehead and is divided into three sections: the dorsol lateral section, the interior orbital section, and the cingulate gyrus. The prefrontal cortex is the most evolved part of the brain and is responsible for time management, impulse control, organization, and critical thinking. Those that experience problems with the prefrontal cortex have a limited attention span, distractibility, lack of perseverance, impulse control problems, chronic lateness, poor time management, disorganization, procrastination, unavailability of emotions, misperceptions, poor judgment, difficulty learning from experience, short-term memory problems, and social and test anxiety. [44]

It seems apparent that these difficulties would preclude one from excelling in school. Amen states that those with problems of the prefrontal cortex experience difficulties with the retrieval of information and concentration and have trouble activating this part of the brain under stress, even if they have adequately prepared for a test. This also applies to social situations as decreased functioning of the prefrontal cortex causes one to lose a train of thought during conversation. When people with ADD try to concentrate, prefrontal cortex activity *decreases* rather than increases. This limited attention span and distractibility prevents one from completing projects. Parents, teachers, and supervisors often apply pressure in hopes of improvement, but this is not effective. Amen advises using praise and encouragement in lieu of demands to improve performance. [45]

People with ADD experience great difficulty sustaining attention for mundane activities because of decreased prefrontal cortex function. Hyperactivity, restlessness, and humming are ways to stimulate an underactive prefrontal cortex. It is interesting to note that Amen states that people with ADD unconsciously seek conflict as a way to stimulate their prefrontal cortex and, hence, become addicted to turmoil. If one cannot seek turmoil in an external environment, often one seeks it within oneself. This often prompts one to pursue a fast-paced life, highly stimulating behaviors (e.g., sky diving), or to use drugs and alcohol. Teachers, parents, and work supervisors commonly respond using negative reinforcement (i.e., yelling or lecturing). The negative behavior often decreases if one responds to this behavior *softly.* Amen believes that this may help to break the addiction to turmoil. However, this addiction to turmoil often leads to repeated mistakes. [46]

The prefrontal cortex allows one to feel and express emotions. The limbic system controls mood and the libido. The prefrontal cortex facilitates the activities of the limbic system and helps to translate emotions into expressions of love, passion, or hate. Underactivity or damage to this part of the brain often leads to a decreased ability to express thoughts and feelings. Perhaps this is why so many artists, writers, and musicians are only capable of expressing their emotions through paintings, poetry, or songs. On a positive note, those who repress their emotions may be capable of producing extensive works of art, poetry, or music.

Those with ADD often struggle with impulse control and decision making. Poorly thought out decisions relate to impulsive behavior. People with ADD often want an immediate solution and act without the necessary forethought. The prefrontal cortex is also the part of the brain that helps one to learn from mistakes. Those with decreased prefrontal cortex function have a tendency to consistently make the *same* mistakes and not learn from them. How many times have you heard a teacher or parent say to a child, "How many times do I have to tell you not to do this?" Every time I move or impulsively quit or take a job, my mother yells in exasperation, "Don't you learn? Didn't you think about this?" It is an inability to think through the consequences of behavior and this affects our social interactions and daily activities: poor choices selecting a mate, interacting with customers, dealing with defiant children, spending money needlessly, and driving recklessly. SPECT studies revealed significant increased activity in the prefrontal cortex with Adderall medication. [47]

Dr. Barry Jacobs at Princeton University believes that serotonin's primary task is to facilitate motor (muscle) activity. Compulsive, repetitive movement likely boosts serotonin. Hence, exercise and activity is highly beneficial for those with ADHD and will produce positive effects. Experiential learning, such as environmental education, employs movement, thus, according to this theory, boosting levels of serotonin. Dr. Jacobs's study showed that chronic exercise doubles not only brain serotonin levels but also serotonin activity in the cerebral cortex. The effects lasted for weeks after training ceased. Sleep deprivation can produce a 20 percent decrease in brain serotonin. Depriving animals of rapid eye movement (REM) sleep, the sleep stage in which serotonin neurons are almost completely at rest, caused increased appetite, sexual and locomotor activity, and fighting.[48]

Other proposed theories of the causes of ADHD include environmental toxins, prenatal factors, and food additives. One-third of children with lead poisoning do display ADHD symptoms. However, refining one's diet alleviates ADHD symptoms in only 5 percent of children, and most people with ADHD do not have a history of prenatal problems. Most likely, ADHD is complex, and the etiology remains unknown. It may be a conglomeration of factors, but physiological theories seem to prevail.

One may find empirical studies that demonstrate the effectiveness of stimulant medication such as methylphenidate (Ritalin). Although 50 percent of children with ADHD exhibit positive changes in academic performance as a function of methylphenidate, 20 to 30 percent of children with ADHD do not respond positively to the drug.[49] In one study, twenty-four six- to twelve-year-old boys, out of a total of eighty-four children, participated in an eight-week summer treatment program for ADHD children. Results revealed that methylphenidate improved academic functioning, but on a short-term basis. Behavior modification did not have an effect on children's academic work; completion of and accuracy on the academic tasks were no better with behavior modification than in regular classroom conditions.[50]

The behavioral effects of medication do not persist beyond four to five hours from the point of ingestion, with the exception of sustained-release medication. In addition, increased heart rates have been observed. Therefore, children with ADHD who manifest Tourette's syndrome, high levels of anxiety, numerous fears, and psychosomatic complaints are not considered good candidates for psychostimulant medication. Another disadvantage of medication is what is referred to as psychostimulant rebound. This is the behavioral deterioration that occurs in late afternoon or evening after an earlier dosage. Symptoms of psychostimulant rebound include increased restlessness and inattentive behavior, elevated levels of hostility, and/or emotional lability.

State-dependent learning may occur with the administration of psychostimulant rebound. Studies attempt to clarify if information learned may be retrieved or recalled only when the person is on medication. There are no conclusions, but performance is facilitated while on medication. In children, some studies indicate that methylphenidate does suppress growth. Psychosis, involving visual and tactile hallucinations, has also emerged in rare cases. Disturbance in thought processes and the development of delusional beliefs have also been observed. Studies of long-term efficacy have concluded that there is no evidence that medicinal treatment yields better academic outcomes, more positive peer relations, or less antisocial behavior.

Two major classes of antidepressants have been used in the treatment of ADHD: tricyclic antidepressants (TCAs) and monoamine oxidase inhibitors (MAOIs). Studies have concluded that MAOIs produce immediate, clinically significant behavioral improvement, similar to the effects of psychostimulants. However, the major disadvantage of MAOIs is the dietary restrictions. Foods high in tyramine, which is found in many foods, must be avoided. Also, MAOIs are contraindicated for impulsive behavior, one of the hallmark symptoms of ADHD!

TCAs immediately provoke changes in attention and impulse control, although it takes weeks to produce an antidepressant effect compared to psychostimulant medications. Tricyclics produce behavioral improvements mainly in the evening due to a longer half-life. As opposed to psychostimulants, sleep disruption is less likely, and improvements have been noted in mood and self-esteem. Tricyclics may be a good alternative for those ADHD children exhibiting anxiety and depression. However, tachycardia is a serious side effect (a heartbeat greater than 100 beats per minute). Less serious side effects include skin rash, dry mouth, constipation, and drowsiness. Furthermore, upon evaluation of long-term efficacy, attentional effects may diminish over time.

Ritalin is a Schedule II drug, a category that includes amphetamines, cocaine, morphine, opium, and barbiturates. Ritalin, Dexedrine, and the tricyclics may have detrimental long-term effects on the immune system and the body in general. These drugs affect the basal ganglia and the corpus striatum, brain areas responsible for increased motor control and sense of time. In addition, they alter levels of neurotransmitters in the brain. In particular, positron-emission tomography (PET) scan studies have shown a marked decrease in dopamine, a neurotransmitter that facilitates movement. Dopamine projects axonal impulses into the prefrontal areas of the frontal lobe, as well as to subcortical structures, including the basal ganglia. As Ritalin increases dopamine production, the brain decreases the amount of its own natural production.[51]

I will admit that, out of desperation, I first started taking Ritalin for premed courses when I was contemplating medical school. It was as if a suffocating fog had lifted from my life. For the first time, I stopped watching the clock in class, playing with my pen, and tapping my feet. I heard every word of the lecture and took copious notes. I felt as if I were a sailboat on a placid lake, instead of a buoy bobbing up and down on erratic ocean waves. Ritalin, although a stimulant, has a paradoxical effect in people with ADHD; it produces a calming effect.

However, Ritalin transformed my personality and it was if another person possessed my body, a person I did not know. One becomes accustomed to acting and being treated in a particular way for many years. Suddenly, a dark veil is lifted and it is as if one experiences daylight for the first time, bright rays of sunshine. Initially, it is intriguing, but out of fear, it is safer to retreat back into what is familiar. One learns to nurture depression, and in a tragic way, cling to it . . . unfortunately, it often culminates in a wealth of creativity. Perhaps this is not so unfortunate, as some of the greatest pieces of music, art, and literature are derived from the depths of despair and one questions abandoning depression for fear of losing or relinquishing certain aspects of creativity.

After extensive research and scrutinizing the studies on Ritalin and other stimulant drugs, I have spent the past five years struggling to find solutions and treatments that do not include traditional psychotherapy and medication. My current daily regimen includes a multivitamin, 75 milligrams of B_6, one flaxseed oil capsule (an omega-3 fatty acid; see Chapter 4), exercise (farming, swimming, yoga, biking, kayaking, or hiking), and meditation.

Ritalin and other psychostimulant medications are a bandage, a quick fix. In our society we seek to satisfy our needs immediately, regardless of the consequences, and drugs offer that possibility. Much of their popularity has to do with the greed of pharmaceutical companies. Three full-page advertisements for stimulant medications recently appeared in *Ladies' Home Journal*. Celltech Pharmaceuticals, the British maker of Metadate CD, touts its panacea as "one dose covers his ADHD for the whole school day." Shire Pharmaceuticals, a British company that makes Adderall, also advertises directly to consumers but does not name the products. Instead, ads request interested readers to call a toll-free number. McNeil Consumer Healthcare, the maker of Concerta, runs a sixty-second commercial on cable television networks such as the Discovery Channel and A&E.[52]

Unfortunately, in a capitalistic society, money takes precedence over education. Sales of stimulant drugs soared to $758 million last year, an increase of 13 percent from 1999. The top three stimulant medications were Adderall, Ritalin, and Concerta. Adderall alone had sales of $248.8 million dollars, and physicians wrote 6.1 million prescriptions for Adderall. In 2000, doctors wrote almost 20 million monthly prescriptions for stimulants. How many of these physicians are knowledgeable about ADD/ADHD? The majority of these prescriptions were written for children, especially boys.[53]

Schools have played into the hands of the pharmaceutical industry, as school psychologists, teachers, and principals are telling parents to medicate their children. If parents fail to comply, they are often blamed for negligence or an inability to control their children. The problem has become so prevalent that state legislators are moving to prevent schools from recommending or requiring that parents put their children on medication. Recently, Minnesota became the first state to bar schools and child protection agencies from telling parents to medicate their children for disorders such as ADD/ADHD. Similar bills have been introduced in Arizona, New Jersey, New York, Utah, and Wisconsin. Connecticut will surpass this by implementing a new law that prohibits any school staff member from discussing drug treatments with a parent.[54]

Although this partially addresses the rampant distribution of medication, it does not resolve the primary problem. It is similar to treating an addiction, a secondary problem, but not treating the primary problem of depression. What about changing curricula and traditional classroom settings and then generating studies to evaluate the efficacy? Should we expend the time and money for education now, or spend it in the future on health problems related to detrimental side effects of these drugs? It seems this is a "penny-wise pound-foolish" choice.

The alternatives to traditional psychotherapy that I propose as an antidote for ADD/ADHD include environmental education, spirituality (nature and religious), community service, meditation, yoga, tai chi, art, poetry, music, and organic farming/food. The common denominator is that these activities are all interactive and hands-on. Furthermore, as previously mentioned, they are *progressive*. They also involve creativity. The benefits of what I refer to as "progressive and experiential" therapy are numerous: reduction of depression and anger; control of mood swings and addictive behavior; improvement of focus, concentration, and social skills; increased self-esteem; decreased impulsive behavior; and identification of new vocational/avocational interests.

These experiential therapies are a cognitive-behavioral approach. Psychotherapy could be enhanced by the integration of the powerful techniques of behaviorism, and the experiential methods of cognitive therapies.[55] Cognition refers to all mental activities associated with thinking, knowing, and remembering; examples of cognitive abilities include memory, creativity, and intelligence. Aaron Beck developed cognitive therapy and attributed difficulties to faulty, negative thinking and self-statements. One of the major premises of cognitive therapy is that thinking helps behavior.[56] Cognitive therapies assume that our feelings and responses to events are strongly influenced by our thinking. Cognitive therapists teach new, constructive ways of thinking and thus try to restructure thought processes.

Behavior therapy applies learning principles to eliminate undesirable behavior. For example, if one suffers from depression, then the premise is to eliminate the disturbing thoughts and maladaptive behavior and replace them with constructive ways of thinking and behaving. This includes providing one with new direction. Social work focuses on a strengths-assessment approach, wherein the therapist emphasizes the client's strengths. An emphasis on one's strengths empowers the client to believe that he or she is capable of making choices and decisions and assumes client competence.[57] However, emphasizing one's strengths is not enough; a therapist or teacher must encourage and nurture these strengths by identifying new interests or assisting in the pursuit of current interests. These proposed therapies might also function as an approach to anger management, as frustration, addiction, and aggression can be positively channeled into activities requiring a great expenditure of energy.

In a paradoxical way, restlessness provided me with some stability and a desire to seek a calling in life. After my return from California, I worked at a summer camp but walked out after a few weeks, deeply frustrated. A personality conflict quickly emerged with the director, a former accountant and totalitarian who consistently reprimanded me. On a positive note, it encouraged my yearning to spend more time immersed in nature, allowing time for reflective thought. Desperate for another job, I called PACT one day from a pay phone to find out if it was not too late to work as a summer intern. I was informed that they were short of interns and I would be welcomed with open arms, with the stipulation that I would resume classes in the fall.

Chapter 2

The Web of Deception

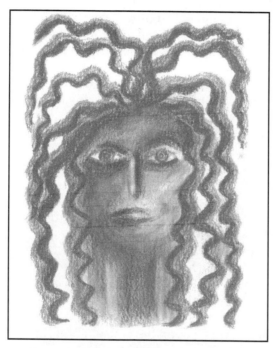

If a man have not order within him,
He cannot spread order about him.

Confucius

It is almost 7 p.m. and I am standing with Carl, my supervisor, amidst pure pandemonium in the city emergency room. It is my first bedside consultation, an extensive, confidential drug and alcohol history, treatment planning, and DSM-IV diagnosis (*Diagnostic and Statistical Manual of Mental Disorders,* Fourth Edition, a classification system designed to assist clinicians in treatment planning). Carl actually does the consultation while I observe. Apparently, they utilize the medical model: see one, do one, teach one. I feel like a charlatan, trying to appear competent by donning a long, white lab coat and arming myself with a clipboard and pocket DSM, my summer tan fading fast in the pallid lighting of the hospital.

We get a brief social background from Mr. Leone, the thirty-one-year-old patient. Carl explains that the patient's physician refers anyone entering the hospital with a possible drug- or alcohol-related illness to our program, so that we can make treatment recommendations to the patient and physician. This particular patient is an intravenous (IV) drug user addicted to heroin and HIV positive.

"When did you first begin using heroin, Mr. Leone?" Carl prompts.

Mr. Leone grimaces in pain, contorting his facial features.

"Cramping?" Carl asks.

"Yeah, right here." He points to his abdomen.

"That's from the withdrawal. What's happening is that your intestinal tone is returning to normal. Opioids cause intestinal tone to increase and intestinal spasm."

"I don't care what it is, man; it hurts like a son of a bitch."

"Yeah, I know. Lucky for you, you won't die from withdrawal. But if you keep shooting, you will."

"Hmph, tell me about it. I ain't going through this again."

"How old were you when you first tried heroin?"

He grimaces again. "Ow . . . um, I don't know, twenty? You expect me to remember that far back? I can't even remember what I ate this morning."

Carl scribbles something on the consultation form.

"Did you shoot at first or snort?"

"Snorted."

"How much?"

"Whew, you're asking too many questions. Got me?"

"Every day? Weekends?"

"I dunno . . . weekends."

"Any other drugs?"

"Nah, some pot here or there."

"When did you start?"

"About thirteen."

"How much?"

"Maybe a joint with my friends after school."

"How much do you smoke now?"

"Not too much—a joint on weekends. Man, I'm trying to stop chasing that damn dragon, you know what I'm saying?"

Carl nods, writing furiously.

"When did you start using heroin regularly?"

"A couple years ago."

"IV only now?"

"Yeah . . . that's how I got the disease from my ex."

Carl ignores the comment, nodding as if this is routine, which, of course, as I will learn, it is.

"How much are you shooting now?"

"Dunno . . . "

"Uh-huh. Any blackouts, when you couldn't recall certain things?"

"Yeah, used to happen all the time, man. I'd wake up somewhere and had no clue how I got there."

"Any other withdrawal symptoms in the past, other than abdominal cramping, like nausea, vomiting?"

"Yeah . . . I feel like I got the flu somethin' bad, puking all day."

"Uh-huh, and do you think you have tolerance . . . do you need more to get the same high or do you just have less of a high with the same amount?"

"Yeah, I got tolerance."

"OK . . . negative consequences . . . any legal problems because of heroin?"

"Did some time in ninety-four for dealing."

"How long?"

"Eighteen long months. I ain't never going back there."

"Any family problems because of heroin? Your chart says you're not married."

"Well, would you talk to someone who gave you the disease? Haven't talked to my ex in a year. My stepdad died from AIDS, and I ain't seen my real father since the bastard left us when I was ten. My ma's got AIDS, but she's doin' okay."

"Any money problems because of heroin?"

"Well, if you call not having any money a problem, I'd say it is."

"OK . . . any other medical problems?"

Mr. Leone shakes his head.

"Any prior drug treatment?"

"Um . . . they made us go to AA in prison."

"Okay, family history . . . parents or siblings with drug or alcohol problems?"

"My stepdad was a junkie all his life; I don't know about my real dad, and my brother snorts coke."

"Okay, Mr. Leone, that's about all the information I need." He slams the chart shut for effect to conclude the end of the consultation.

"My advice to you would be to think about stopping immediately, given the nature of your health at this time. You'll be detoxed here in the hospital, and once you get out, there are a couple of community outpatient agencies that will treat you without insurance. Have you ever thought about methadone?"

"What, you want me to get hooked on somethin' else?"

"I see what you're saying, but methadone is a lower dosage to help with the withdrawal symptoms, then get you off the heroin."

Mr. Leone shakes his head. "I'll think about it, but, you know, what's the use? Too late, you know?"

"It's never too late. Protease inhibitors are working miracles for some. . . . Have you heard of the cocktail?"

"Are you paying for it?" he asks, glaring at Carl.

"You can get on Medicaid and start going to a clinic and get yourself cleaned up."

"I'll think about it."

"Hey, it's your choice. Do you have any questions?"

"Yeah, can you call a nurse to give me some more Demerol?"

"Ah, the miracle drug." Carl turns to me.

"Thanks for your time, Mr. Leone."

"Thanks," I echo. We walk out of the cubicle and return to the nurse's station to write up the consult for the chart. Carl glances at his watch.

"C'mon, I'll teach you how to review the lab tests."

"Sure," I agree. I've been here almost ten hours, but it has gone by in the blink of an eye. Everything about the hospital mesmerizes me: the technology, the activity, the unpredictability, and the daily ethical dilemmas. Earlier today, I watched a gastroenterologist perform an endoscopy and biopsy a cyst in the esophageal tract. It fascinated me, but after a while, the dehumanization bothered me. The doctor took little notice of the patient, an elderly man drugged up with Demerol and periodically choking on the tube. He was only one of several endoscopies scheduled for the day.

Carl breaks through my thoughts. "Grab a seat," he says and opens a chart.

"OK, our main concerns are the LFTs, or liver function tests, GGTP (Gamma-glutamyl Transpeptidase), SGOT (Serum Glutamic Oxaloacetic Transaminase), SGPT (Serum Glutamic Pyruvic Transaminase) that measure hepatic enzymes. MCV is mean corpuscular volume, the average volume of a red blood cell, and the normal range is eighty to ninety. A high MCV is greater than one hundred, usually common in heavy drinkers; about one-third of drinkers have elevated MCVs. Microcytic cells are small, normacytic is normal, and macrocytic is large. In alcoholics, the platelet count is the first to respond. Over time, the MCV decreases when the drinking stops and bone marrow recovers."

I am fascinated. "How long does that take?"

He shrugs. "A while . . . depends, can be months. Elevated LFTs are usually from alcohol, although drugs or hepatitis can cause LFTs to increase, but the increase means something is wrong with the liver. When the SGOT is higher than the SGPT that means alcohol-induced liver disease. OK, enough lecture. Go try one."

"Me?"

He shrugs. "How else do you expect to learn?"

I love the consults and eagerly run around the hospital, often staying late and attending medical lectures. Medicine and physiology fascinate me, and I seriously contemplate medical school in the coming months. After a while, I am afflicted with medical student syndrome: I definitely suffer from social phobia, perhaps am mildly bipolar one week, with occasionally a schizophrenic symptom or two. However, these tend to surface after I have pulled an all-nighter to write a paper.

Staff meetings are weekly and last two hours. The first hour is group supervision where anyone can discuss a particular client with the rest of the staff. Our outpatient clients are generally working class from the surrounding community, and in addition to drug and alcohol addiction, they struggle with homosexuality, borderline personality disorder, and bipolar and histrionic personality disorders to name a few. Many have a history of incarceration.

The second hour is devoted to intakes. Every clinician is assigned a random intake when a client seeks initial treatment. Every new client's case is presented to the rest of the staff, including a complete drug and alcohol social history, diagnosis, and treatment recommendations. New students always keep the DSM within reach for quick consultation during meetings. Sometimes when the diagnosis is ambiguous, I watch the room in awe. As if reacting to the starter gun at a race, all the graduate students frantically fish around in bags for the pocket-sized DSM, hurriedly skim through pages, and turn to consult one another on the specific distinguishing criteria.

For example, it is generally easy to distinguish between alcohol abuse and dependence, but sometimes there is a fine line. Dependence is defined as three or more of seven criteria occurring at any time during a twelve-month period. Some of the criteria include tolerance; withdrawal; reduction of or abstinence from social, occupational, or recreational activities; drinking longer than intended; and persistent desire or unsuccessful attempts to cut down or control use. If tolerance or withdrawal is present, then physical dependence is also diagnosed. Abuse is defined as meeting one or more criteria within a twelve-month period, such as failing to meet role obligations at work or school, legal problems, or social problems.

During the intakes, clients are assigned for individual and group counseling. Every week, each clinician eagerly waits to pounce on the latest case. Sometimes I feel as if I'm at an auction—one client going once . . . twice . . . sold, for sixteen weeks of cognitive-behavioral therapy. I procrastinate and do not extend myself, but it inevitably happens, and I am assigned my first case. Ryan is a twenty-one-year-old white male with a history of incarceration for possession and distribution of heroin and is currently on probation. One of my colleagues hands me his file.

"Good luck," he says.

I smile weakly.

I call Ryan later that afternoon to schedule our first session. He slurs his words over the phone and explains that he is still in withdrawal and is trying to catch up on his sleep. His girlfriend, also a heroin addict, has run away to New York and is go-go dancing at night. She was recently raped one night on the way home from work. On that note, we schedule a session for that week.

Two days later, I meet Ryan. He is scrawny, about 5'8", and sports a buzz cut and two menacing tattoos on his biceps—one of a skull, the other a dragon. However, it is his eyes that really scare me. They are dark and steely, and he looks at everything intensely, including me. I am slightly apprehensive, maybe a little more. I position myself near the door, especially after he casually describes in cool detail the shanks he's fashioned in juvenile detention and the inmate he stabbed.

During our first session, I concentrate on establishing a rapport and building trust, although I know it will be a long road. He gazes at the ceiling and talks about his addiction to heroin. I can't help but glance at his arms, the pale skin revealing the remnants of track marks.

"Some days," he says, looking up at the ceiling, "I'd say, God, please let me stop after this bag, just one more fucking bag." He stops and fixes his gaze on me. There is no book in any library or class lecture that prepares you for these situations. My mind quickly races through the recent literature I've read and discussions in staff meetings on coping with cravings and urges. Ryan takes a deep breath and laughs.

"And I never thought I'd be here, sitting in some drug counselor's office." Drug counselor? I'm just someone who wrote an essay and fooled a graduate committee, someone with more identity issues than a chameleon. Who am I to dole out advice? I gulp some air.

"Well, the first seventy-two hours are the most difficult, as you know. Aside from all your withdrawal symptoms, you're going to experience a lot of cravings and urges that you'll learn how to ride out. And it will get easier." I do not even recognize my own voice; I sound professional and competent, but inside I tremble with fear and uncertainty. I pull a sheet of paper from my notebook.

"Let's do a decisional balance. It's similar to a list of pros and cons. Sometimes it helps to see things in black-and-white and to have it for future reference. Make a list of the advantages and disadvantages of continuing to use heroin. Over in this column, list the advantages and disadvantages of not using heroin."[1,2]

I hand him a pen and he scrawls a few phrases in each block, taps the pen impatiently, and then writes some more.

"Okay, I'm done." He pushes the paper toward me.

I read out loud. "Benefits of not using . . . girlfriend will stop using. It's interesting that you list only that as a benefit. What about for yourself? Your health, saving money, things like that?"

He shrugs. "I know, I know, I gotta take care of myself, I've been with this girl for seven years. She's my life; I have to take care of her. She looks up to me, and if I stop using, she will."

"Do you really think she will? It sounds as if she's had a tougher time quitting than you have."

"Yeah, she can't go more than four days without doing it. I can stop for months. Maybe I should just kill her. Then I know she'll be safe, and I won't waste any more sleep worrying about that stupid girl."

I am stunned for a minute and then attempt to resume a professional attitude. "Do you seriously think about that?"

"Well, it'd make my life easier. Nobody'd know. I'd just walk up behind her in New York, pull her in an alley, and slice her. No one would miss her. Her stepfather's in California and she hates him. Her mother's dead."

I fumble around for a minute. I'm not sure if this is for shock value, or if there is some truth to this. After all, he does have a violent history. "What if you did get caught? What would the rest of your life be like? You'd be locked away and never have the opportunity to talk to her again."

"I guess." We continue to discuss the rest of the decisional balance, and I bring up the session in group supervision the following week. Everyone seems interested and has some advice to offer.

"You need to evaluate for homicidal ideation. Has he talked about this before? Does he have a plan?" one student contributes.

"Well, somewhat. He's talked about stabbing her in New York. Do I ask him or let him bring it up again? And when do I take him seriously?" We had recently studied confidentiality and the famous Tarasoff case in my law class; the case involved a psychologist who was indicted on charges that he failed to exercise his duty to warn and protect a potential victim. Under New Jersey statute, a duty to warn and protect is incurred when a patient communicates to a practitioner a threat of imminent, serious physical violence against a readily identifiable individual or against himself or herself and a reasonable professional believes the patient intends to carry out the threat. The civil immunity act protects professionals who breach confidentiality under such circumstances.[3]

Dr. Rotgers casually folds his arms, as if he's heard this many times and, of course, he has. "See if it comes up again. Then we'll discuss it." Fortunately, the issue does not surface again, but still it invokes some anxiety in me.

The next week, Ryan calls to inform me that Shanna, his girlfriend, has returned and is temporarily living with him. He wants to know if he can bring her in, and I readily agree. He sounds positive on the phone and informs me that exercise is elevating his mood. I am anxious but excited about the impending session that night.

Seven o'clock arrives soon enough, and I settle into an office, slap the obligatory "Do Not Disturb" sign on the door, and shuffle some papers. Ten minutes later, I hear a girl's voice in the hallway. I stand up to peer out the doorway. Shanna towers over me, leggy and anorexic in appearance. She has long, jet-black hair with a flower tucked behind one ear. Her skin is strikingly pale and dark circles outline her puffy eyes, giving her an owl-like appearance. Fishnet stockings cover her legs and a black miniskirt just conceals the tops of her thighs. Ryan looks annoyed as we sit down, and it is evident that they've been arguing. She begins to cry almost instantly, and I hand her the requisite tissue box.

"Thanks," she says softly and quietly sniffles.

"How are you doing?" I ask her.

She shrugs. "OK. I guess Ryan told you everything."

I nod but do not offer anything in case there are some missing pieces. Ryan immediately jumps in.

"She's using again—that's what she's doing."

"I'm trying to stop," she says, the tears flowing again.

"Bullshit. I can stop. Why can't you? She's got no willpower." He directs this last comment toward me.

"Well, it hasn't been easy. I can't stay with you, and all my friends do it."

"So get out of there!" he demands.

"I can't. I need the money, and it's close to work."

"Yeah, great job, ain't it. Men slobbering all over you."

"I need the money, Ryan."

"There's other jobs. Get a waitress job. You don't have to take your clothes off for that. You don't see me strippin' and dancin' on tables. Go get a respectable job if you think I'm gonna stick around."

She jumps out of her chair. "I told you I'm trying, and it doesn't help when you yell at me." She opens the door and runs down the hall, hopefully only to the bathroom. They came together on the bus, so she most likely won't leave. Wow, we're off to a great first session!

"She'll probably go smoke," he says, clearly frustrated.

"I really do believe she's trying," I say.

"Yeah, but I'm telling you, she's weak. That girl's got no willpower."

"Well, you can help her by getting her through the initial cravings you went through. She doesn't have a car, so that's good. Stay with her at all times and find out what will help distract her most during a craving. Ask her to tell you when she wants to get high. But it's important for you to encourage her and support her . . . congratulate her each day she's straight. Remind her of all the positive consequences you've experienced. Better sleep, exercise, good mood. Look how far you've come in such a short period of time."

"Yeah, I have," he says, smiling for the first time.

As we continue to discuss communication strategies, I glance at the clock.

"Why don't you go find Shanna and ask her to come back. In the meantime, I'll call around and try to locate an inpatient facility with an open bed."

He agrees, and I start flipping through the directories. I make a list of facilities and spend the next fifteen minutes on the phone. Finally, I locate a hospital for indigents that will detox her. I am exasperated to experience firsthand the lack of available detox facilities.

Shanna and Ryan walk back in, and Shanna wipes her tear-stained cheeks.

"Shanna, I found an inpatient facility for you and you don't need insurance." The first step is to ensure her safety and allow her to detox in a supervised setting.

"I think once you get through the next few days, which will be tough, Ryan really wants to help you. You have a good support system."

She sniffles. "I know, and I will go."

"Good." We all smile, relieved, as if a weight has been lifted, although this is only the beginning, the first steps of a long journey. We discuss the facility; I give them directions and end the session. Although I feel a sense of accomplishment, I worry whether she will follow through.

My hunch is correct. Ryan calls the next day to tell me he and Shanna have broken up, and she has moved back to New York.

"I did everything I could. It's just that she's been a part of me for seven years. How are you supposed to let that go?" Just wondering the same thing, I want to say.

"It will be hard, I understand. I also agree that you've done everything you can. But for the time being, you need to hope that whatever you've done or said will stay with her. It's out of your control now and you have to keep moving forward. Think of everything you've gained. You've gotten a job, you're exercising, and you're saving money. Don't let that go."

"Yeah, I know." He sighs heavily and is quiet.

* * *

Addiction is considered a comorbid disorder of ADD/ADHD, a dual diagnosis often rampant among artists, writers, and musicians. There is conflicting evidence over whether a diagnosis of ADHD indicates a risk of developing a substance use disorder (SUD). Some studies indicate that adolescents and adults with ADHD are at high risk for developing a SUD. Approximately 50 percent of adults with ADHD have a history of psychoactive substance use disorder (PSUD) and a history of ADHD has been found in 22 to 71 percent of substance-abusing adults.[4] Another study concluded that adults with ADHD are more likely to have SUD than adults without ADHD.[5] Other researchers also found that those with ADHD of childhood onset persisting into adulthood had a twofold risk for PSUD. Among subjects with an alcohol-use disorder, ADHD significantly increased the risk for subsequent drug abuse or dependence.[6]

However, in many of these studies, a comorbid diagnosis of conduct disorder (CD) or antisocial personality disorder (ASPD) was also present.[7] It has also been hypothesized that SUD is more likely to occur among individuals with the hyperactive subtype of ADHD, although more studies are warranted to examine the relationships between subtypes of ADHD and later substance use.[8] Furthermore, critics of these studies contend that these studies may not be conclusive for a number of reasons. One, untrained clinicians may not use screening instruments such as the Wender Utah Rating Scale and the ADHD Behavior Checklist for Adults. Two, screening instruments should not be exclusively relied on for a diagnosis as it is not uncommon for patients with SUD to complain of inattentiveness, restlessness, problems with organization, and impulsivity once they begin to use drugs or alcohol. It is crucial that a diagnosis of ADD/ADHD be made during a period of drug abstinence. And three, it is often difficult to differentiate between ADHD, major depression, and bipolar illness. For instance, *structure* often reduces distractibility and excessive talkativeness among patients with ADHD, whereas structure does not typically improve manic symptoms. ADHD is also characterized by an early onset; mood and anxiety disorders typically have a later onset.[9] The majority of these studies also represent males with ADD/ADHD. There are many women with undiagnosed cases of ADD/ADHD because their symptoms are disregarded in schools.

Nevertheless, many adolescents and adults have undiagnosed ADHD and do not seek treatment until an addiction takes precedence over their lives. As a result, this often leads to a misdiagnosis and treatment for substance abuse or dependence, which often masks the true symptoms of ADD/ADHD. In one study, 33 percent of alcoholics seeking treatment had adult ADHD. [10] In another study, a childhood history of ADHD was present in 34.9 percent of cocaine abusers, although none had a *current* diagnosis.[11]

Often people with ADD/ADHD may unconsciously try to restore levels of neurotransmitters or escape from the depression or mood swings they often experience, although the "self-medication" hypothesis has been challenged.[12] It is interesting to note that adults diagnosed with ADHD often use psychostimulants such as amphetamines and cocaine that have similar effects to the stimulant medication used to treat childhood ADHD.[13] Cocaine abusers report improvements in their inattentiveness and impulsivity.[14] From my counseling and personal experiences, addiction is often secondary to depression and other symptoms of ADHD. Once the primary symptoms of ADD/ADHD are addressed, the addictive behavior often diminishes.

However, even after the ADD/ADHD symptoms are treated, I believe that addiction may continue to be a concern for some. It is alluring to be high or inebriated; there is an irresistible attraction to be immersed in a haze and to be alienated from pain is preferable at times to reality. Managing ADD/ADHD can be a lifelong journey and treatment for symptoms is not a miraculous, overnight cure. Overcoming the psychological wounds that ADD/ADHD leaves may take years and it is often tempting to resort to former negative coping skills during tumultuous times. Thus, the "stages of change" model, as described in the following paragraphs, may apply in these situations. Many people struggle with the initial diagnosis of ADHD and perhaps cycle through the similar stages of bereavement: denial, anger, grief, bargaining, and acceptance. Many individuals encounter difficulty with medication compliance and traditional psychotherapy, and perhaps this is partly due to the rebellious personality trait that many people with ADD/ADHD possess. Therefore, harm reduction and moderation management, as described in the following pages, may initially be an effective approach to treating addiction problems, *concurrent* with treatment for ADD/ADHD.

Irrefutably, we need to implement *early intervention* programs and perhaps some of the approaches that I suggest in this book would be effective as such. The successful identification and early treatment of ADHD might alter the progression of PSUD.[15] Economically, early intervention programs in schools to diagnose and treat ADHD will decrease the financial burden to society in the hopes of avoiding a later substance use disorder. However, the reality is that 14 million children under the age of twenty-two years old had no health insurance coverage in 1999. Families rely exclusively on publicly funded services and uninsured youth receive care for *acute* symptoms only, which again only addresses the addiction and not the ADD/ADHD. Outpatient services are covered for a brief time. Medicaid does cover inpatient and outpatient substance abuse and mental health services, but reimbursement rates for health providers are low, deterring many from offering these services. It is also difficult to recruit professionals trained in addictions medicine.[16] Many turn to self-help organizations such as Alcoholics Anonymous (AA) or Narcotics Anonymous (NA), but again, the majority of people running these groups are not trained to recognize the primary symptoms of ADD/ADHD.

The current remedies for addressing these problems are screening instruments, medication, and psychotherapy. There are two widely used drug and alcohol screening instruments for adults seeking a clinical evaluation for ADD/ADHD: the Drug Abuse Screening Test (DAST) and the Alcohol Use Disorders Identification Test (AUDIT). The DAST is a twenty-eight-item instrument that assesses drug-related consequences of use and abuse. In addition, it detects past and current drug abuse. The AUDIT is a ten-item questionnaire developed in conjunction with a World Health Organization (WHO) project to detect harmful alcohol consumption. The AUDIT only identifies current alcohol abuse. There are no data on the reliability and validity of these tests.[17]

Stimulant medication has been documented in several studies to decrease ADHD symptoms and drug abuse or dependence. One study found that methylphenidate not only reduced ADHD symptoms, but also cocaine use in individuals diagnosed with ADHD and cocaine dependence. Another study of adolescents found that subjects with ADHD who received medication were much less likely than the non-medicated ADHD subjects to develop a SUD.[18] Another study indicated that patients with a SUD had greater improvement in their ADHD symptoms with methylphenidate than patients without a SUD.[19] Hence, it may be hypothesized based on these particular studies that substance abuse may be a consequence of ADD/ ADHD and that these individuals were perhaps self-medicating.

However, there are no studies to evaluate the efficacy of pharmacologic or nonpharmacologic treatment for patients with a SUD and ADHD. Furthermore, there are "no standard nonpharmacologic treatments for adult ADHD."[20] Various treatment options show promise, but there are few programs available. Substance abuse treatment programs are experimenting with two approaches referred to as nodal link mapping and sensory integration that may be beneficial for treating substance abuse among patients with ADHD. Nodal link mapping utilizes spatial-verbal displays to visually demonstrate interrelationships between ideas, feelings, facts, and experiences. Sensory integration seeks to group stimuli in an organized fashion. A combination of cognitive-behavioral therapy and medication can also be successful with patients with ADHD and SUD.[21] Again, the treatment approaches that I suggest in this book are a cognitive-behavioral approach. Interestingly, there is evidence that patients with a SUD are likely to improve if engaged in an ongoing, *structured* treatment and medication should be considered a supplement to treatment.[22]

In Chapter 7, I propose that yoga be considered as a treatment for ADHD, as well as those diagnosed with ADHD and a co-existing SUD. A number of studies have found yoga to be effective in addiction treatment; considering that many in substance abuse treatment centers have a history of ADHD, it may therefore be a beneficial therapy for those with ADHD. One study of a methadone clinic discovered that yoga was just as effective as traditional psychodynamic therapy and reduced cravings, anxiety, and fear. Dopamine is elevated in the basal ganglia of the brain when drugs are introduced to the body. The brain begins to crave that dopamine surge and this is one physiological explanation of the struggle to abstain from drug use. Yoga and meditation may dampen dopamine activity in the basal ganglia, which in turn inhibits cravings and emotional states that trigger drug use.[23]

If one can increase self-esteem, alleviate depression, and identify new avocational/vocational interests through alternative therapies, one can be taught how to channel one's addictive behaviors into positive outlets such as exercise and extracurricular activities. This redirection of addictive behavior may lead to inventions, completing marathons, or writing books. Sometimes one has traveled so far down the path of destruction that it may seem impossible to find the way back. If someone intervenes at a crucial time with concrete, pragmatic therapies, or if the addict reads a particular book, it may be equivalent to giving the addict a compass for the first time.

This is similar to the concept of self-efficacy proposed by Albert Bandura. Self-efficacy is confidence in one's ability to cope with a specific task or challenge. Immersion in nature, in the form of wilderness experiences or gardening, for example, may provide one with a challenge. If one can conquer new challenges, perhaps this enhances self-efficacy and, therefore, self-esteem, leading to abstinence or reduction of drug and alcohol use. Self-efficacy has been central in various treatment approaches.[24]

James Prochaska and Carlo DiClemente proposed a theory referred to as "stages of change," one which we were made well acquainted with at PACT, and which holds relevance for those with ADD/ADHD. In the stages of change model, each individual passes through five stages: precontemplation, contemplation, preparation, action, and maintenance.

Precontemplation is the stage where one does not acknowledge a problem, although families, friends, and co-workers may threaten to terminate relationships or employment. It is only under feelings of coercion that one seeks help, and one often has no intention of changing behavior.

In the contemplation stage, one acknowledges a problem but is not committed to taking action. This stage can last for long periods of time; in one study, 200 smokers stayed in the contemplation stage for two years. Furthermore, one may struggle with the pros and cons of continued use, focusing more intently on the positive aspects of continuing use.[25]

Preparation is the stage where individuals form a concrete plan to assume action in the near future and will make small changes, such as smoking five fewer cigarettes a day.

During the action stage, one modifies behavior, environment, or experiences to accomplish the objectives. However, a consistent change in behavior made one day must last for six months. It appears that an internal locus of control manifests in these individuals, as many believe they have the autonomy, or self-efficacy, to make changes in their lives. Individuals in this stage also increasingly rely on the support and understanding from relationships. This is where family, friends, and religious, spiritual, or other organizations can lend support.

In the maintenance stage, one works to prevent relapse for an indeterminate period of time.

One may cycle through these stages several times before maintaining abstinence. Most individuals regress to an earlier stage and become easily discouraged. However, the majority of relapsers progress once again to the contemplation or preparation stage. The stages of change theory offers an explanation of the struggles faced by those suffering from addiction, but, as with most traditional treatment programs, it does not provide adequate treatment options to reduce the risk of relapse and help individuals to progress more quickly through these stages.

In an effort to move beyond traditional treatment approaches to achieve better success and reduce the rate of relapse, PACT utilized harm reduction, "a public health alternative to the moral/criminal and disease models of drug use and addiction."[26] Harm reduction is an incremental and gradual approach that aims to reduce alcohol and drug use in a nonconfrontational manner, while still recognizing abstinence as an ideal outcome, for example, condom distribution and syringe exchange programs. Indisputably, harm reduction should be applied to working with people with ADD/ADHD, and the alternative therapies presented in this book are analogous to a harm reduction approach.

A major principle of harm reduction theory is that abstinence is *not required* as a stipulation of treatment, as is the case in traditional treatment programs. The majority of clients in four addiction studies (as high as 84 percent) *chose* abstinence as a goal when *offered a choice*. The imposition of treatment goals often leads to poor treatment outcomes.

Harm reduction empowers clients and provides them with the capability of making their own decisions about alcohol and drug use, rather than viewing them as "powerless" and mandating abstinence. The therapist merely serves as a facilitator and helps the client work on achievable drinking goals. Furthermore, therapists who maintain a positive expectancy for client outcomes evoke self-fulfilling prophecies.[27] Therefore, in the context of helping those with ADD/ADHD, educators who maintain a positive expectancy for their students may elicit self-fulfilling prophecies as well.

In addition to harm reduction, moderation management of alcohol consumption is another alternative, depending on such factors as existing medical problems, younger age, lower severity of dependence on alcohol, and social and economic stability. Moderate drinking is possible for those who are capable of abstinence for a period of time, typically thirty days. This helps one to lower tolerance, to identify urges and cravings in particular situations, and to recognize an ability to think more clearly. A variety of guidelines exist that help to define a moderate drinking plan. This includes four standard drinks (equivalent to ten ounces of beer, four ounces of table wine, and one ounce of 100-proof spirits) per day for males, a maximum of three standard drinks per day for females, and a maximum of five drinking days per week. A client agrees to stay within these limits over a duration of time in the context of safe drinking situations. Progress is measured through self-monitoring and the development of alternative coping strategies. If a client fails to achieve these goals, the therapist works with the client to modify them.[28]

* * *

In the fall, I am assigned another challenging client. A change has occurred within; I am more attentive and focused. Andy is forty-two, has a long history of drug abuse, and is now attempting to abstain from seven years of drinking binges. He has recently lost his license for a DWI, as well as his restaurant due to alcohol problems. During our second week of sessions, I am ten minutes late. I rush in, try to catch my breath, and find a key for a vacant office. Andy is waiting in a chair in the hallway, glaring at me. He stomps behind me into the office, grabs a chair, and sits down.

"You're late," he states accusingly.

He instantly puts me on the defense. I hold my tongue and try to be polite. "Yeah, I'm sorry. There was a lot of traffic." Granted, I probably had overslept.

"Well, I'm not late. I'm here on time and I expect the same of you."

I want to start screaming at him about the thousands of dollars in loans I have accumulated so that I can be here to counsel him, my four demanding classes, and my own personal problems. Instead, somehow I muster some patience and fight my instincts to shout an expletive or two, storm out of the office, and slam the door. Guess this is as good a time as any to develop some conflict resolution skills. Anxiety ties my stomach in knots, and I take a deep breath.

"Andy, I am really sorry and I have not ever been late before. It won't happen again. So . . . what's going on with you? Did something happen in the last couple days?"

He sighs, releasing a long, deep breath. His face falls. "It's just been a bad week. I spent all day at the DMV. I can't get my license back for another six months. I waited an hour for the bus in the rain, missed the second one, and my hip is killing me." (He previously had hip replacement surgery.) "I just woke up angry." He sighs again. "I'm sorry for yelling at you. It wasn't you."

"No worries. I'm sorry you're having a hard time." We talk the rest of the session, and I encourage him to play his bass again and to stop by the library on his bus route to find some cooking books. Andy had once played the bass guitar but abandoned it for many years in favor of alcohol. He is smiling by the conclusion of our session.

"Thanks. I felt like coming in here before and ripping this place apart, throwing the chair across the room. I do feel a lot better." He stands up, shakes my hand, and leaves. I am astounded at the outcome of this session and proud that I have successfully resolved a conflict. If I had reacted in my usual manner, I probably would have lost my internship as well as a client for our program.

The next session, Andy brings me a recipe for vegetarian chili that he had previously concocted at his restaurant. I am touched.

"I've been doing some cooking," he says, proudly. "And you'll be happy to know I found my bass and stopped at the library the other day on the way home. I actually got a library card and took out some books."

"That's great. You seem in good spirits today."

He nods. "Yeah, not too bad."

I assign "homework" for the first time and ask him to keep a journal of his cravings, complete a decisional balance, and practice anger management skills (a collaborative learning experience) and relaxation techniques. He returns all the writing assignments in following sessions, and I am quite surprised, but happy. For the first time in my life, I feel I have truly helped someone. Furthermore, he has remained sober as of the initial session.

I see Andy twice a week for sessions and that, in itself, presents a challenge. I discuss this with my direct supervisor, Patrice.

"Why is that so hard for you?" she asks me one morning.

"I don't know. I wanted to ask you that myself. It's very intense. It almost feels like a relationship. Don't you feel that way?"

She shakes her head and a puzzled expression crosses her face. In psychology jargon, perhaps this is some countertransference on my part. I am forced to confront my own struggles; there is no escape. I do not voice this thought but continue along another line of reasoning.

"Actually, I've taken a much more active role. I really care about his progress. He even returns his assignments, follows my advice, and never misses a session. He's maintained sobriety for one month, the first time in seven years. It amazes me!"

"Why does it amaze you?"

"I don't know. It's extremely rewarding that I've played such a role in someone's life."

"There's nothing more rewarding than that," Patrice says, smiling.

By the end of the semester, it is almost hard to terminate and transfer Andy to Patrice. She has agreed to accept him as a client, and I carefully highlight my progress notes, emphasizing his direct needs and goals. Andy hugs me good-bye upon the conclusion of our last session, taking me by surprise. I will really miss him. As he is walking down the hall, he turns around.

"Hey, come visit my restaurant someday. I'm going to open another one."

"Can't wait." I smile and wave good-bye.

*   *   *

So, perhaps one successfully manages one's drinking or substance use. However, the prevailing depression or sense of purposelessness may still exist. The solution lies in progressive therapy. People with addictive personalities can learn to channel this excessive energy into other outlets that require great concentration. Success in occupations such as painting, writing, music, and farming are contingent upon having an addictive personality; one must expend great amounts of energy and persistence, working intensely for extended periods of time. I find that those with addictive personalities can accomplish these tasks and completely immerse themselves with an energy of which others are not capable. Being challenged by and deeply absorbed in one of these fields takes precedence over hangovers, and time is no longer taken for granted. Finding one's calling or a new path in life can be a *progressive* form of therapy. The following chapters suggest alternatives to traditional treatment options that are progressive in nature and applicable to those suffering from ADD/ADHD. These alternatives revolve around nature and discovering new vocations and avocations that give one a sense of purpose, a sense of belonging, and a sense of accomplishment.

Chapter 3

The Eternal Maze

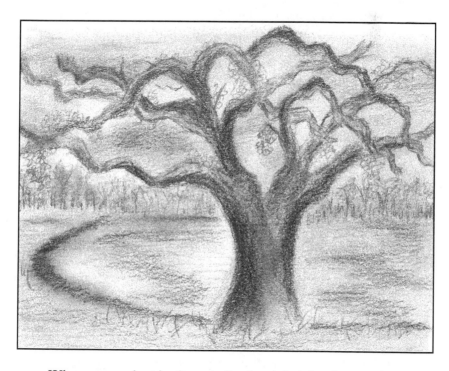

When we are lost in the woods, the sight of a signpost is a great matter. He who first sees it cries, "Look!" The whole party gathers round and stares. But when we have found the road and are passing signposts every few miles, we shall not stop and stare.

C. S. Lewis

Under overcast and gray skies, I trekked through the forest to seek out my tree, my first assignment. Raindrops trickled down my hood and coated my eyelashes. I wiped them away and squinted at the fine mist that had settled. I continued on the trail until I found it, a lone tree that ceased to grow, surrounded by pines, spruces, oaks, and maples. I studied it for a while, droplets of rain falling from the foliage onto my paper. I pulled a clipboard from my backpack and covered the paper with a plastic bag. I glanced around the forest at the acres of trees surrounding me, feeling happily secluded. I clutched the board and scrawled a poem, holding the pen sideways under the plastic bag:

> a patchwork of decaying bark
> covered in moss green
> and intricate scars
> carved by various inhabitants
> wraps itself around
> a willowy spindle for a trunk
> only to diverge
> as two lone branches . . .
> remnants of wilting leaves
> curl from lack of nourishment
> and cling to a protruding limb . . .

Rain broke through the thin canopy of trees and it seemed a good time to retreat. I followed the trail to the edge of the forest and what I thought would lead back to the nature center. I came to a fork that did not strike me as familiar but chose a path I believed would lead me in the correct direction. I walked another fifteen minutes and became slightly alarmed. For some inexplicable reason, I often continue walking or driving for miles in strange places without turning back, until I succeed in getting myself truly lost. Perhaps it is a subconscious wish.

Miles of wheat and holly bushes lined the trails and hazy, blue mountains dotted the horizon. A maze of trails branched out in every direction. I was trapped in an analogy, representing my life. In a couple of hours, darkness would fall. Could they find me? I studied the bushes and wild milkweed, but I was not confident enough in my knowledge of edible plants to gather an adequate dinner. I decided to plod along, perhaps on paths to destinations unknown.

Rich, fertile soil and furrowed fields converged in the distance. I walked through interminable rows of tomato plants and could not resist the urge to steal a Brandywine tomato, biting into its tantalizing skin. When I reached the end of the row, I spotted a greenhouse. One lone farm worker, who appeared of Spanish descent, watered plants.

"Do you know where the nature center is?"

He looked at me, perplexed, and shook his head.

"No hablo inglés."

As I feared. I scrambled around in my head to piece together some broken Spanish.

"Dónde está . . . el centre de naturel?"

He nodded, understanding.

"No," he said and shrugged.

Fantastic. We could communicate, but I still could not get directions.

"Dónde está el teléfono?" I asked in desperation.

He smiled, nodding. "Ah, si, señorita," he said, motioning for me to follow him. He led the way to an old stone house and inside to a small office.

"Muchas, muchas gracias," I said relieved.

"De nada, señorita," he replied and walked out.

Embarrassed, I hoped I wasn't the first and only intern lost when sent out on a simple assignment! However, this was an 800-acre nature preserve. Rick, the assistant education director, laughed, not expecting to hear from me on a telephone. After the humiliation settled, I agreed he could pick me up, the little forlorn figure I was, enveloped in an oversized raincoat. I looked like a drowned rat, abandoned on the side of the road. A few minutes later, car tires crunched along the gravel road and Rick drove up. He smiled and opened the door.

"Thanks," I said sheepishly.

He laughed again. "No problem!"

We zoomed down the farm road in what I now recognized as the direction back to the nature center. My mind drifted back to our staff training, an intense two-week crash course in ecology. One day I hiked a different trail, identifying wildflowers, such as foxglove, beard-tongue, and yarrow. Later, I researched wildflowers for their medicinal uses. Another day I mulched the new butterfly garden and planted milkweed, dill, parsley, broccoli, and cauliflower to attract monarch caterpillars. During an introduction to forest ecology, we trampled through the forest and studied leaves to identify trees. I vividly recall the day, brilliant summer sunlight filtering down through the foliage.

We sat on a carpet of pine needles, inhaling their scent wafting through the air, while Jeff, the environmental education director, and Rick helped us distinguish between round and pointed lobes of white and red oak leaves, respectively. The intricate network of xylem and phloem tissues created a beautiful webbed appearance. We learned silly, but memorable, acronyms, such as MADHORSE, representing indigenous East Coast trees that have opposite branching: maples, ashes, dogwoods, and horse chestnuts. We identified alternate branching trees, simple and compound leaves, pinnately and palmately compound leaves, smooth and dentate leaf edges. We twirled conifer needles between our fingers to identify them as flat (firs and hemlocks), square (spruces), or "packages" of two or more (pines). We scrutinized bark, seeking characteristics such as furrowed ridges. For instance, red oaks typically have grayish-brown, red-tinged bark and wide furrows between ridges.

Identifying trees became a favorite pastime. Shagbark hickories and sugar maples captivated my attention, and I could not claim a favorite, admiring each for its own unique beauty. The shagbark hickory stands majestically proud, its trunk striving to reach the sky, "shagging" its bark after forty years. The bark of the sugar maples intrigued me, the stark contrasts of dark and light gray swirling together into knots. I studied dendrology and the many benefits trees and shrubs provide: carbon dioxide sequestration (the conversion of carbon dioxide to oxygen); energy conservation by reducing temperatures; prevention of wind and water erosion; renewable resources for paper, food, and wood products; and replenishment of groundwater aquifers. I incorporated my newfound love into paintings, collecting brilliant crimson maple leaves in the fall and portraying them in a painted collage on canvas, superimposed over faint yellow beech leaves and a green background.

Down at the pond, wading knee deep in fresh water, we tested the water for pH, ammonia, and nitrogen levels and seined the brook to study crayfish, darters, and other life. Droplets splashed on my legs and the sun sparkled on the water, scattering prisms of scintillating light. We concluded training late Friday afternoon and collapsed on the grass. We begged Rick to let us go home. He laughed and yelled to Jeff, who ran over barefoot, never one to bother with shoes in the summer.

"They said they want to go home," he moaned, mimicking our tired voices.

"Well, should we let them? Can they tell me the difference between a red oak and a white oak leaf?"

"Who cares!" someone shouted.

"You will when someone asks you!" Jeff yelled back.

Justin, lying in the grass, raised his head and mumbled, "Red oak leaf has pointed lobes, white oak has rounded."

Jeff nodded his approval. "A star pupil. OK, go home, get some sleep this weekend. It may be the last opportunity for a while."

"Yippee," we grumbled and staggered to our cars.

The following Monday morning, I began teaching the myriad of information I managed to learn to a group of children ranging from preschool to middle school. I'd never taught before, and this presented a new challenge. I had just finished graduate school two weeks before and found this opportunity, an internship teaching environmental education. I'd wanted a new challenge, and it had presented itself.

Every morning, I scrambled out of bed, scrounged through my dresser, threw on some shorts and a ratty T-shirt, and pulled my hair back in a ponytail. Breathless, I dashed in and, with the other teacher-naturalist, grabbed bug nets, field guides, a first aid kit, and "bug boxes" for an insect safari or seine nets and water chemistry kits for a pond/stream program. We raced over to the main office, a 200-year-old white, rambling farmhouse, then collapsed into rocking chairs on the front porch to wait for the morning's group. Various groups of kids from local YMCA camps arrived daily for one morning class.

For a stream ecology class, we hiked the Four Seasons Trail to Stony Brook Stream, prodding thirty or so kids along. My favorite group was the inner-city kids. Mesmerized and wide-eyed, they would huddle together, fearful of the ominous woods. It astonished me to hear some of them mention they had never seen a tree. Once we arrived at the stream, we waded through the babbling brook, seining with the net to catch crayfish, tadpoles, and darters. For insect safaris, we'd "sweep" the vast, open fields with bug nets and capture them in bug jars and boxes. The dogbane beetle mesmerized me with its shell of iridescent red and blue. Considering I had somewhat of a bug phobia, I managed to relay enough enthusiasm that a group of girls emerged from the woods after a class chanting, "We love bugs! We love bugs!" That was a measure of success.

I led hikes and learned to identify wild, edible plants such as milkweed and dogbane. I spent the last three weeks painting a fifteen-foot wall mural depicting the effects of water quality on the mountains, farmland, a housing development, and factories. I taught outside in the morning, then rushed inside to paint feverishly all afternoon, covering the walls with vivid hues of cobalt and cerulean blue, viridian green, and cadmium yellow. Stony Brook also hosted monthly folk music concerts under the vast starry night sky, as well as occasional poetry gatherings.

And to think that I almost quit in the first two weeks. I had no patience or tolerance for boredom and consistently made impulsive decisions, usually based on a fleeting moment. Jeff convinced me to stay.

"Just open your heart," he said. And I did. By the end of the summer, I'd contracted poison ivy and fatigue from the extreme heat of this particular summer. But to have the opportunity to open these kids' eyes to the infinite treasures of nature far surpassed my aches and moans. I recalled Jeff's words in my head from the first week of staff training: "Some people come back ten years later and tell me this was the best summer of their life." Ha, I thought at the time. Indisputably, it was one of the best summers I ever had. I had spent hours blazing over trails in the woods with my mountain bike, seeking that adrenaline rush, but never once stopped to identify a tree. It is astonishing what you can find in your own backyard. I've searched high and low for fulfillment in my travels, suffering from a perpetual case of wanderlust.

I stumbled into environmental education by accident and it changed the direction of my life. One afternoon during my second-year graduate-school internship at an alternative school, I was thumbing through a recent issue of *Teaching Tolerance* magazine. An article on therapeutic gardening intrigued me, and I raced to the vice principal's office to share the article. She shared my enthusiasm and showed me the way to a closet filled with gardening tools and seeds. A horticulture teacher had initiated a garden, but no one had pursued it once she left the position.

Dissatisfied and frustrated with traditional therapy and education, I knew I had to implement an alternative solution. These kids, the majority diagnosed with ADD/ADHD, had no more desire than I did to sit in the confines of a stuffy classroom and discuss their feelings. We were interminably met with a stream of obscenities and airborne objects.

Two weeks later, on a morning early in March, we began our "therapeutic" garden. Although the temperature hovered around thirty-two degrees and snow flurries drifted through the air, twelve students diligently raked and dug up the turf, preparing the earth for the first planting season. My friend David offered to help me start the garden. He worked to build a compost bin with some of the students, who eagerly asked questions and sawed lumber.

Throughout my internship and working with these students in the context of psychotherapy groups, I had never seen such enthusiasm or attention to any task. We continued to work in the garden, took a trip to a nearby farm to learn chores, painted a mural of an oak tree in my office, and cleaned up abandoned lots. During this farm trip, several inner-city students expressed interest in working on a farm. These trips served to identify new vocational interests never previously expressed simply because they lacked the environmental exposure! Suddenly, some of these kids smiled and revealed information about their childhoods. Carlos, a seventeen-year-old, worked consistently next to me and described his dreams of starting his own landscaping company. Until then, we'd never exchanged a word. Trina, typically irritable and confrontational, smiled at me and enthusiastically described growing and canning tomatoes with her mother.

When we started the community garden, I had an insatiable desire to learn everything about gardening. I had never had positive learning experiences sitting in a classroom nor felt the desire to learn from a textbook. But all that changed. The fresh air stimulated and provided me with excessive energy to burn. I had spent every waking moment of my childhood outside, preferably on a bike or in my beloved tree house. Although my mother had grown up on a farm and periodically dragged us to the remote cornfields of Iowa, I could not tell you how to plant a seed. But I did recall vivid memories of picking raspberries for my great-aunt to bake a raspberry pie and of running through the cornfields with my brother. David fueled my desire to learn farming and environmental education and opened the door to a whole new world for me.

At Rutgers, I became involved with campus environmental organizations for land preservation. To my surprise, a local paper published an editorial I wrote. My friend Scott asked me to work with him on a campaign to build bike lanes between campuses. We created student surveys and attended city hall meetings. I loved to spark controversy and found an outlet for channeling repressed anger, rebellion, and frustration into something positive. Activism permits, and even encourages, such characteristics. David brought me to Green Party meetings, a nonviolent, third-party political organization that focuses on promoting social justice, ecological wisdom, and environmental issues. It further ignited my interest in activism, particularly in farmland preservation. I met people with whom I shared common values and interests and eventually presented a paper on the Green Party to my Human Behavior and the Social Environment class.

Artists, writers, and musicians, often diagnosed with ADD, can use their paintings, poems, and songs to express their convictions and advocate for solutions. Farmland preservation is of particular interest to me, but it is only one example of innumerable environmental and social problems. Other prevalent issues today include water quality, sustainable community forestry, world hunger, welfare, housing, adoption, and family planning. Teachers can play critical roles in invoking an interest in activism by teaching students to write letters to Congress and local newspapers, bringing their attention to current events, and perhaps even taking students to a town hall meeting. For instance, recently in my ecology class, we discussed Clinton's proposed ban on commercial logging and we wrote letters in support and sent them to Congress. In art class, we constructed "zero circles," a nationwide art movement initiated by an environmental artist to support the ban. We trekked through the woods, seeking any natural materials to form a circle, photographed it, and mailed it to this particular artist. Using his art, he intended to elicit support from artists across the nation in an attempt to arouse media attention and thus gain public support for the ban on logging.

I started to bike with the local New Brunswick chapter of Critical Mass, an organization initially formed in San Francisco to advocate for sustainable transportation, encouraging people to use bicycles in lieu of cars. We blocked the streets of New Brunswick, yelling, "Use your legs, not your engines!" I ran around campus, sometimes in the rain, tagging bikes with slips of paper advertising for the rides.

* * *

The early infusion of environmental education (EE) into general and "alternative" educational curricula may serve as an intervention for those children with ADHD. Environmental education is a broad concept. From my experiences, it may involve community gardening, stream or forest ecology, entomology—essentially anything about nature that one can teach. EE incorporates math, history, social studies, science, creative writing, English, music, poetry, journalism, activism, psychology, and political science. As a formal definition, one researcher defined EE as a discipline that "focuses on human-environmental relationships encompassing cultural, political, ethical, philosophical and aesthetic interpretations and that demands a problem-solving, inquiring, action-oriented approach."[1] Others define environmental knowledge as a student's ability to understand and evaluate the impact of society on the ecosystem, as well as comprehend the origins, implications, and consequences of problems resulting from people's intrusion upon the ecosystem.

Other ecopsychologists define the field of ecopsychology as the application of ecological insight to the practice of psychotherapy and the study of the interrelationships among all forms of life. Traditional psychotherapy emphasizes the interaction among humans and does not take into account the impact of surrounding factors. Psychology is the study of the psyche or soul. Ecopsychology may be viewed as the study of the psyche or soul in relation to circumstance.

Based on my research, there appear to be psychological, social, and perhaps long-term economic benefits for our natural resources as children develop a respect and appreciation for their environment. Psychological benefits include an increase in self-esteem, a sense of accomplishment, and identification of new vocational or avocational interests. This may also be considered a strengths assessment approach. Social benefits include building group cohesion, improving communication skills, encouraging an exchange of ideas among peers, and generating practical solutions to problems.

Environmental educators hypothesize "that it is best to learn about the natural environment in the natural environment. Therefore, experiential education in nature is seen as being more effective than classroom learning."[2] David Orr, professor at Oberlin College and founder of the Meadowcreek Project, views all education as environmental education and teaches students that they are a part of the natural world.[3] One study surveyed 172 boards of education in Ontario and concluded that students benefit from direct experience in nature.[4] Roszak believes that "nature's diversity keeps the human imagination alive, the creative processes animated, the tolerance for difference possible."[5] Hippocrates looked to nature to find the wisdom of healing. In all cultures, nature teaches us the rhythm of balance. A small garden teaches the cycles of life: time to plant, grow, harvest, decay, and regenerate.

In the eternal classic *Walden,* Henry David Thoreau speaks words of wisdom—wisdom that seems to elude every generation:

> How could youths better learn to live than by at once trying the experiment of living? Methinks this would exercise their minds as much as mathematics. If I wished a boy to know something about the arts and sciences, for instance, I would not pursue the common course, which is merely to send him into the neighborhood of some professor, where any thing is professed and practised but the art of life;—to survey the world through a telescope or a microscope, and never with his natural eye; to study chemistry, and not learn how his bread is made, or mechanics, and not learn how it is earned; to discover new satellites to Neptune, and not detect the motes in his eyes, or to what vagabond he is a satellite himself; or to be devoured by the monsters that swarm all around him, while contemplating the monsters in a drop of vinegar. Which would have advanced the most at the end of a month—the boy who had made his own jackknife from the ore which he had dug and smelted, reading as much as would be necessary for this—or the boy who had attended lectures on metallurgy at the Institute in the mean while, and had received a Rodgers' penknife from his father? . . . Even the poor student studies and is taught only political economy, while the economy of living which is synonymous with philosophy is not even sincerely professed in our colleges.[6]

I spent two years teaching at a Zen Buddhist alternative high school. Students were high school-aged adolescents who had been expelled from public school or were completely disillusioned with traditional education; the majority carried diagnoses of ADD/ADHD. The staff had the unique opportunity to teach their passions and develop their own curriculum. I developed and taught art, ecology, and agriculture curricula (see appendixes). Other staff members taught yoga, writing, woodworking, a Zen martial art, blacksmithing, and foreign languages, as well as the academic subjects required for a high school diploma. The school emphasized community; students and staff cooked, ate, and cleaned up together. Each morning, students sat for a twenty-minute meditation followed by a brief discussion focusing on various topics such as compassion, mindfulness, and the benefits of meditation.

During forest ecology, we stomped through the forest for wild, edible plants and researched their culinary and medicinal uses. This component of horticulture may encourage a student to pursue a career as a horticulturalist, chef, or naturopath. On hikes, I discussed the inner layers of a tree, maple sugaring, and tree identification. Forest ecology introduces students to the benefits of trees and encourages their participation in preservation and activism. During art, we sat in the farm fields to paint the distant mountains or traveled to a nearby river to paint reflections. I recently explained to an amused student that whatever we draw or paint is a reflection of our subconscious. In a landscape painting class at the Pennsylvania Academy of Fine Art one summer, I painted an eerie magnolia tree, its branches forming an intricate maze, perhaps symbolizing the confusion I experienced as to what direction in life to pursue. I encourage students to use their imagination, draw or paint in the abstract, and study something from different angles to see what piques their curiosity.

Recently, we embarked on our first overnight camping trip to a nearby state forest. Despite the rain and temperatures in the fifties, it was a great success. We hiked five miles around the lake before sunset, and I spent the time talking to Lauren. Quite insightful, she spoke a great deal about ADD and frustrations with constant distractions. As we walked, she cried out, "Look—an orange salamander!" She gleefully picked it up, her eyes wide with wonder, cupping it gently in her palm.

"See, one of the good things about ADD is that you see things that others don't. Most people are always in a hurry or are just not observant. That's a benefit that may help you in a career someday. Maybe you'll be a naturalist, reporter, or artist," I pointed out. "Those are all professions that require great observational skills."

Lauren and I continued along, picking up salamanders and examining them, as well as an array of wildflowers. As we plodded along, the sun set quickly and a fine mist enveloped the forest. We had underestimated the time it would take to complete the trail. Fortunately, another staff member gave Lauren a flashlight, although the small beam of light barely penetrated the darkness. We walked for another half hour before we spotted a light up on a hill. Excited, we charged through the woods, but the light elicited disappointment, revealing an outhouse. I knew it was an error in judgment to leave the trail. Momentarily, darkness prevailed, disorienting us, and we could not find the trail again. My heart pounded slightly, a hint of panic, although one would think I'd be accustomed to getting lost. The forest was desolate; apparently no one else had the desire to camp in this weather. Suddenly, Will, one of my co-workers, spotted a road and a directory. After carefully scrutinizing the map tacked to the bulletin board, we decided to follow the road back to the park office. Although the office was closed, I knew the general direction from there back to the campsite.

Fatigued, we trudged up the hill. Headlights startled us, beaming through the darkness from the top of the hill. I quickly glanced at Sherry, another staff member, and we sprinted up the hill. Gasping for breath, we stopped. A family was packing their car. I explained that we were from a school and had lost the way to our campsite. I hoped they would offer a ride to the office, but they merely pointed us in the right direction. We hardly appeared threatening, but our bedraggled appearance may have raised some doubt in their minds. The other members of our group lagged behind us. Disappointed, we walked away. Suddenly, we heard drums in the distance. We had brought conga drums and had drummed around the campfire earlier in the day. It was Robby, another staff member, and Jarod, a student. We yelled across the lake at the top of our lungs and heard a faint return holler.

"Drum louder!" we screamed.

The beat of the drums increased in intensity, and we followed the sound. Someone spotted a clearing in the woods and a wide trail along the lake. A quick unanimous decision and we ventured along. Out of nowhere, two lanterns illuminated the trail in front of us, swinging eerily, suspended in the darkness. Robby and Jarod emerged behind them. We all hugged, happily reunited, and simultaneously explained our adventure. Back at the campsite, warm in front of a crackling fire, Lauren turned to me and said, "Even though I was a little scared when we were lost, it was an adventure . . . something to tell my grandchildren." It was worth it. Jarod entertained us with bad jokes for the next hour, but we wound up convulsing into fits of laughter. Finally, exhausted, we crawled into our tents. I snuggled into my sleeping bag, dressed in layers of clothing, and fell into a deep slumber.

The next morning, Robby caught bass with Jarod and Lauren. I sat with them on the dock, watching the water lap along the edges of the shore. Brilliant white birches lined the perimeter of the lake, some curving out over the water. Wispy shrouds of mist hung over the lake and patches of blue sky crept out between the clouds. After an hour, we returned to the campsite to grill the bass, Jarod and Lauren boasting of their catch of the day. Lauren and I tested the lake for pH, determining it was good at 6.5. She loved the water ecology kit I bought for a class and wanted to purchase her own. Reluctantly, we walked back to the campsite to leave, as we had to be back by late afternoon. Tired and silly, we laughed and listened to radio stations blaring bad music on the way home. We provided the entertainment at the next staff meeting, jokes abounding about our sense of direction, or lack thereof. I admitted spatial abilities and planning were not my strengths.

In the fall, we embarked on another camping trip. Despite rain and cold temperatures once again, we found a cabin on the premises to rent. Once settled, several students went to fish with Robby and I hiked in the rain with two students, the brilliant fallen foliage of glistening amber and crimson red maple leaves blanketing our path.

These camping trips served to build group cohesion and community. Students who previously had difficulty working together in class diligently worked together to build a campfire, collecting wood and exchanging ideas on how to start a fire, or offered help to pitch a tent. Spontaneous therapy sessions occurred, and one of these happened in my bunk one night with a student, who talked openly for hours until bleary-eyed. The conversation gradually evolved from family life to teaching to existentialism.

*   *   *

Wilderness experiences are mandatory to make appropriate environmental decisions. Such experiences open us to our feelings, a deeper sense of caring and compassion. The Redcliff Ascent Outdoor Therapy Program in Utah offers an intensive, minimalist wilderness therapy program to "build character and restore self-esteem" away from music, television, and cell phones. Participants hike, build campfires, prepare food, dig latrines, and pursue high school course work. The students engage in daily periods of introspection; psychiatrists and psychologists visit once a week to measure progress. Students de-velop values of respect, compassion, and increased self-esteem. Red-cliff is one solution when increasing numbers of public schools fail to deal with severe behavioral problems, drug use, and violence. State and local courts also use the programs as an alternative to jail. Pro-gram officials tout Redcliff as the most direct way to save a wayward life.[7]

Those who present the argument that these programs may offer a temporary solution and simply send individuals back to their original environments where they are likely to lapse into past behaviors are incorrect. Many programs instill values that last long beyond the ter-mination of the programs. If a convict learns to garden in prison, he or she is armed with new values and knowledge and may return to his or her environment to transform an abandoned city lot into a bountiful garden that in turn links the community together, provides food and beauty, as well as teaches others to live a sustainable life.

Robert Greenway, an ecopsychologist at Sonoma State University, collected 700 questionnaires about two- to four-week wilderness trips that included fellow professors, graduate students from other departments, local psychotherapists and psychiatrists, and various wilderness leaders. Some of the findings were as follows:

- Of the respondents, 90 percent described an increased sense of aliveness, well-being, and energy.
- Ninety-two percent cited "alone" time as the single most impor-tant experience of the trip.
- "Community" or the fellowship of the group was cited by 80 percent as the third most important experience.
- Seventy-seven percent described a major life change upon re-turn (in personal relationships, employment, housing, or life-style), and 38 percent of those changes held true after five years.
- Ninety percent stated that the experience allowed them to break an addiction (defined very broadly, ranging from nicotine to chocolate and other foods).[8]

The human need for understanding the natural world is as essential as the basic needs humans share with other animals, such as food, air, water, and shelter. Some environmentalists state that the recom-mended approach is to infuse EE into all subject areas and at all educational levels. Perhaps EE needs to be incorporated into Maslow's hierarchy of needs! In particular, community gardening may foster group cohesion, build trust, lend a sense of accomplishment, and increase self-esteem.

Community gardening is one component of EE that can be traced back to the very beginnings of communities and gardens themselves. The word "community" originates from the Latin root *communis,* which means "common." The modern community is defined as people who join together out of a matter of necessity or desire. Community can be any group of people living in the same place bound together by the same government, social class, activities, or interests. The phrase "community garden" has come to mean almost any group of people who garden together in any setting, urban or rural. The exchange of ideas, growth of food, relaxation, and creation all take place within this social context. In the late 1970s, community gardens were established in every state, especially in urban areas.[9]

Community gardens in schools can emphasize cooperation by having students from various ethnic backgrounds with differing skills and abilities work together to create a garden. In the context of a garden or forest, painting or writing, spontaneous conversations develop. This *empowers* an adolescent, granting him or her some measure of control and choice concerning topic of conversation. In such a setting, adolescents do not feel coerced to answer questions. Out of the blue, students may speak of their struggles with depression or addiction or of a family problem. The therapist may immediately learn something, instead of relying on innumerable attempts to elicit information in a formal setting. For instance, I recently counseled a new student who, frustrated during a sporting event, stormed off in the direction of the forest. After a few minutes passed, I checked on him. He sat hunched over, a lone figure by the creek, head down. We discussed some of his past experiences, his hatred of competition and difficulty in making yet one more transition. Suddenly, his eyes widened as he spotted a large ant. He proceeded to tell me that he found ants fascinating because he liked their organization and linear processes.

Another afternoon while sitting on a hill painting the garden, this particular student refused to finish his painting. I sat down next to him and quietly pursued his underlying fears. In a weary voice, he disclosed that he did not want to complete the painting because he would be disappointed, as he had been disappointed in everything else in his life.

"I understand your fears," I said. "But if you don't continue to try, you will never conquer this feeling of disappointment. You could accomplish something great someday, but if you don't try, you'll never know."

"Yes, but I don't want to worry about having expectations and letting myself down," he countered.

"So don't set expectations. Easier said than done, but just keep your mind open and give it your best shot. Disappointment is an inevitable part of life. But sometimes it's the disappointment and failures that encourage us to keep trying, and, eventually, the accomplishments supercede the disappointments."

He appeared contemplative for a minute, then got up and walked away with his painting. I let him go.

The freedom to seek solitude when overly stimulated, either in a classroom or other setting, grants students a degree of autonomy unavailable to them through traditional educational and therapeutic approaches. Traditional therapists may contend that alternative environments are distracting and do not permit controllable conditions. However, I discovered two things that I would not have discovered in a formal office setting. First, this student had an appreciation for entomology and perhaps I could encourage this. Second, I had insight into his cognitive processes and fears, knowledge that would be beneficial to the course of his treatment and my future interactions with him.

Label something as "therapy" and resistance may automatically develop. Freud postulated that resistance was a serious impediment to the therapeutic process. As rebellion is a characteristic trait of most people with ADD, do not expect cooperation! A therapist or teacher who employs an empathic, nonconfrontational approach is more likely to obtain compliant behavior. We are a society that does not understand delay of gratification, and this is evident in the overprescription of such medications as Prozac and Ritalin. Medications are beneficial at times for a brief duration, but they inevitably serve only to mask the symptoms and do not teach one to resolve the underlying problem.

Furthermore, in the context of a community, conflict resolution skills develop as a result of staff and peer feedback. Many teachers working with students with ADD coerce students into resolving a situation immediately. Naturally, in one with ADD, this provokes a rebellious and antithetical response. Learning to resolve conflict happens over time, and it is often on the student's time. If a teacher can relinquish control, the student gains an illusion of control, and the outcome is rewarding to both the educator and the student. Although some researchers discuss resistance as an integrative value in coping and expression of autonomy, do we really need to engage adolescents in any more combative relationships, many of whom have been reared in conflict-ridden households?

Community gardens are not just limited to schools. Adults can find a local community garden and volunteer or start one in their neighborhoods, nursing homes, homeless shelters, or psychiatric hospitals. Anyone can volunteer or intern for a nature center/preserve. It has enriched my life, opened my eyes to the world of ecology, and given me a sense of purpose. It involves constant activity and diversification, which is ideal for someone with ADHD. I volunteered with some AmeriCorps friends working in downtown New Brunswick on Saturday mornings. We dug garden plots for anyone in the community interested in maintaining a garden. People on the street often walked by, looking curiously at ten to fifteen students raking, shoveling, and weeding. Often, their curiosity led them to question our motives, and after learning of the program, many requested plots. This experience built community, initiated interest among community members in growing their own food, and turned a previously vacant lot into a haven of peace and beauty.

Anecdotal evidence from numerous schools suggests that the outdoor environment can help children achieve independence, self-esteem, and social skills—all deficits in children with ADHD. One science teacher related the story of a student who had spent two years in a "behavior" class for fighting. The student was mainstreamed into general education classes only after working on a greenhouse project and then pursued an agricultural program.

In a 1997 study at Virginia Tech, 75 percent of teachers reported frequent improvements in student behavior in the context of a garden as a learning environment.[10] Researchers at Our Lady of the Lake University in San Antonio, Texas, conducted a three-year school garden study (1995-1997) of twelve third-grade classrooms.[11] They found that the self-esteem of students in gardening classrooms increased in year one and remained high during the next two years. Students in gardening classrooms also exhibited a greater increase in awareness of and interest in social concerns (e.g., feeding the hungry) and improved relationships with other students and parents as opposed to students in control classrooms.

Schools with programs for special populations have long known the benefits of teaching horticultural skills to students who are limited physically or mentally. Success with growing plants provides the encouragement that students need to learn new skills and also gives practice in using tools, addressing motor, sensory, and mental deficits.

To illustrate with a personal example, I worked with a nineteen-year-old depressed and drug-addicted adolescent. All the odds were stacked against him; AIDS had claimed his mother's life and his father was incarcerated in prison for life. He lived with a friend's mother. He had recently been caught with a cat tranquilizer known as "Special K" in school and was on the verge of expulsion and criminal charges. The principal intervened and sent him to work on a flower farm across the street. Presently, he is still enrolled in school, completing his senior year, and pursuing a horticultural program at a local technical school.

Cathrine Sneed's Garden Project has helped hardened criminals from the San Bruno, California, jails find a sense of dignity and return to their inner-city communities with vital survival and entrepreneurial skills. Gardening in correctional institutions decreased the recidivism rate in participating facilities by 21 percent in 1996.[12] Recently, I had the opportunity to hear Cathrine speak at the Northeast Organic Farming Association (NOFA) annual conference. An inspiration, she has devoted her life to building a successful horticultural program. She spoke of the financial hardships she endured, but these, she said, could be overcome with a sense of community and support from her enthusiastic staff.

Environmental programs are emerging throughout the country. In *Reclaiming the Commons: Community Farms and Forests in a New England Town,* Brian Donahue, a founder of Land's Sake in 1980, writes about the community gardening program established in Weston, Massachusetts, for middle-school suburban children. "Better to get them out of the classroom and back on the land," he states.[13] At Land's Sake, youths transplant, hoe, and hand-weed crops; stake tomatoes; lay down mulch; and pick, wash, and sell produce on a twenty-five-acre organic farm. Early spring is devoted to tapping maple sugar trees and boiling sap to make sugar. Fall finds the apple cider press crunching apples into sweet cider. The ten-week summer program includes weekly field trips and serving lunch at local homeless shelters in Boston, and as many as 100 children participate each summer. "Parents like their children to get their hands in the soil and learn where their food comes from. . . . Parents love it when the children come home all covered with dirt and so proud of themselves. That's real education," Donahue writes.[14] Participation in the summer program leads to identification of vocational interests. Some of the students eventually pursue careers as farmers, horticulturalists, or natural resource managers.

Food Works, founded in 1988, is a Vermont-based nonprofit educational organization that has developed a school program called Common Roots. The mission of Food Works is to address the social needs of hunger and malnutrition by teaching hands-on gardening skills in public schools. Most important, it is a solution to provide students of all abilities with opportunities for learning experiences and practical applications of knowledge. This educational program covers practical skills in science, social studies, nutrition, math writing, and the arts. Food Works has implemented this program in twelve Vermont public schools and now facilitates curriculum development across the country.

Common Roots offers a three-credit course to equip teachers with horticultural skills and the ability to institute an environmental education program. This program may include indoor and outdoor activities, such as indoor gardens, outdoor historic theme gardens, composting, cooking, and baking. Food Works has also developed Gardens for Learning, a privately funded program to deliver food to children. Students cultivate vegetables and herbs in an organic garden, which may be located on school grounds or optional sites, such as at churches, community housing projects, and trailer parks. This program reinforces cooperative learning, provides nutrition education, and teaches the value of community service.

4-H programs focus on experiential learning, believing that youths will develop knowledge, attitudes, and skills to become competent, caring, and contributing citizens. Community service projects provide active learning interaction between youths and adults and encourage youths to set and accomplish goals. In 1901, Captain E. Miller of Keokuk, Iowa, sponsored a county organization of boys and girls that included officers and educational programs. His plans shaped the teaching tools of today's 4-H programs, including life skills, learning-by-doing projects, group meetings, and exhibits. Today, 4-H offers youths opportunities in communications, leadership, career development, livestock, home improvement, and computer technology. These programs are found in rural and urban areas throughout the world.

Healthy child development depends on healthy interactions with the natural environment. If stimulation is not provided during "critical periods" in early child development, children are at risk for never achieving their potential in certain developmental areas, such as language, social skills, and emotional health. Furthermore, if respect and caring for the natural environment are not formed during early childhood, these attitudes may never develop.

Students learn and retain information when they see it in its proper context. You cannot pick up an oak leaf from a textbook and see its tiny network of xylem and phloem tissues or examine the lobes to determine if it is from a red or white oak. A textbook cannot ever accurately depict the experience of wading in fresh, invigorating streams and sinking your feet into the sandy bottom as you catch crayfish and water insects.

A survey of 225 kindergarten through twelfth grade (K-12) Illinois public-school teachers revealed that 90 percent of the respondents agreed that it was important to integrate EE concepts into their subjects and that teachers should help students develop values and feelings for the environment. Of the respondents, 87 percent agreed that active learning, when utilized in EE, is the most valuable affective domain education method, and 92 percent agreed that cooperative learning is a valuable method. Most important, self-directed learning, case studies, and lectures made up the three least-valued methods.[15]

* * *

After a couple of experiences working on a maple sugar farm in New Hampshire with my friend Scott, talking with maple sugar farmers, and reading *The Amateur Sugar Maker* by Noel Perrin, I decided to try a small-scale version at school. I contacted a maple sugar farm, conveniently adjacent to our school. The owner, Glenn, and his wife, Cindy, maintain a 130-acre farm, tapping trees and selling produce in the summer from their garden. Cindy bakes 600 maple pecan pies during the sapping season for sale at a local school. Glenn built his sugar shack and enthusiastically offered some assistance, lending buckets, spiles (taps for trees), and a four-wheel all-terrain vehicle (ATV). On a brilliant blue day in early March, we trekked up and down snow-covered hills, identifying maple trees and hammering spiles into trees. Initially, I wanted to make a trial run, tap a few trees, and boil sap in the kitchen using a flat pan. This plan quickly disintegrated, as many students could not contain their excitement, running haphazardly from tree to tree and hammering spiles into the bark. We tapped thirty-five maples and stopped there only because we ran out of buckets. When we finished, the forest was a sea of trees adorned with white buckets, some hanging precariously off maples that clung to cliffs overlooking the creek.

In the mornings, Robby and I drove the ATV and a wooden trailer down to the creek with two empty garbage cans and students in tow. We scrambled up the hills, slugging along five-gallon buckets filled to the brim with sap (initially, the sap is 98 percent water and 2 percent sugar). When the snow melted, we slogged through the characteristic mud of March. We dumped our precious collection of sap into thirty-two-gallon garbage cans and then drove it over the bumpy fields back to Glenn's, often with students crouched in the back of the trailer. There, we dumped it into a 125-gallon tank on the back of Glenn's Kubota 2900 tractor to be siphoned up to a 500-gallon tank in the loft of the sugar shack, where a cheesecloth bag filtered out large pieces of debris that may have fallen in the buckets. The sap was then pumped down through pipes to the evaporator, an immense container where the syrup was boiled.

The mishaps began the first week. One morning, Glenn's German shepherd, Dylan, followed us back to school. We assumed he would return home, and we walked down to the kitchen. Suddenly, one of our students burst in and yelled that Dylan had eaten one of our cancer-ridden pet turkeys. It turned out that he had taken a chunk out of its side; it was bleeding profusely and could not withstand the wound. Robby reluctantly agreed to expedite its death, casting a pallor of gloom over the remainder of the afternoon.

One Saturday, Robby, Colin, a student, and I gathered at Glenn's to boil our syrup. On this particular afternoon, Glenn taught me how to drive the Kubota. He stood on the back and encouraged me to drive faster. After a burst of exhilaration, I thrust it into sixth gear and turned back just in time to see Glenn lunge for the bucket as a means of support. I could not contain my laughter and apologized. After he resumed his composure, he laughed as well. I drove for a while, stopping every few minutes for Glenn to collect buckets and dump the sap into the tank. The snow had melted and the tractor plowed through the viscous mud. Thoroughbred horses grazed on the fields, and a flock of sheep (a breed found in the Old Testament known as Old Jacob's) ran around with three deer, one of whom was named Spindle. Spindle begged for our attention, always prancing up to the fence and waiting to be petted. Someone gave Glenn and Cindy Spindle when she was a baby, and Cindy had cared for her during her infancy. We stopped by the barn and Glenn handed me an Old Jacob's lamb to hold. It snuggled against me, and I sunk my fingers into its wool, already thick after only a week. Hesitantly, I gave her back, and Glenn hopped on the tractor to drive through rough terrain. I stood on the back, and we stopped every few minutes to collect and dump buckets.

Over the course of the morning, we collected a few hundred buckets and drove back to the sap house for boiling. Inside, Robby and Colin were stoking the woodstove every five minutes to maintain a 220-degree temperature in the evaporator. When the thermometer reached a measurement of eight bricks, we drew off the boiling sap into a beaker and measured it with a hydrometer for the proper density. At a particular density, we flooded it into a large tin pail and brought it over for filtering. Colin presoaked filters in hot water and then filtered the syrup to be transferred into a large metal pail. Glenn filled a couple glass bottles and handed the job to me. I filled innumerable bottles and then placed them on their sides to seal the tops. This flurry of activity demanded great attention to make sure that everything was working simultaneously.

We worked diligently until the afternoon and then headed out to collect the remaining few hundred buckets. Many might think this a mundane task—not at all. It is meditative; the silence allows one to listen to a robin or two announcing the impending arrival of spring. The fresh air invigorates and the creek waters gurgle and flow. One learns which maples yield greater quantities of sap and how to distinguish the bark of sugar, silver, and red maples. Sugar maples are ideal for tapping, but silvers and reds also yield sap. It is also pleasurable to be in the company of others. One gains a sense of accomplishment and a feeling of living within the seasons, reaping the benefits of a renewable and natural resource. Most of all, nothing compares to the sweet taste of freshly made syrup boiled over a wood-burning stove, lending it a distinctly smoked flavor.

Tapping maples is also conducive to building community. Over the years, Glenn has been featured in several local newspapers, attracting many customers. He often gives group demonstrations to schools and organizations such as Girl and Boy Scout troops. He leaves his shack open twenty-four hours a day for customers, who are always welcome to buy syrup, leaving money in a basket.

Later in the afternoon, we drove back to the sugar shack to dump the last tank. Suddenly, we spotted a police car. We looked at each other in alarm and raced up to the shack. Glenn was standing outside in his overalls, dousing the roof with a bucket of water. A policeman and several volunteer firefighters wandered around, poking through the shack. Someone advised that we stand back. Smoke curled in wisps from the perimeter of the smokestack. Several fire engines came careening up the driveway, sirens wailing, and, suddenly, small flames leaped from the cedar shingles. Two more fire engines arrived on the scene and firefighters jumped down, pulling hoses off their trucks. A steady stream quickly squelched the flames. A few damaged shingles left a gaping hole, but we breathed a sigh of relief for Glenn that the sugar shack had not disintegrated into ash. An exciting conclusion to the day.

Once the days and nights were above freezing, the season concluded, around late March. Ecstatically, we collected and boiled seven gallons of syrup. Robby volunteered extra time after work and on weekends to attain this amount. One tree can yield up to ten gallons of sap; however, it takes between forty and fifty gallons to boil one gallon of syrup. In art class, students painted maple leaves on masonite boards for the syrup bottles. Will scanned them into his computer and printed them out onto labels to achieve a miniature painting. We affixed the labels to the bottles, and Buffy, who teaches cooking, took them to various health food stores in the community to sell the syrup for a yearbook fund-raiser. In self-government class, students designed a syrup committee and appointed a treasurer to monitor sales. Despite some initial chaos, a few missed classes, and some mishaps, it was a fantastic time.

This is an ideal example of a true interdisciplinary curriculum, involving chemistry (boiling), math (tracking sales), business skills, art, forest ecology, and physical education. Socially, it built community through a group effort and identified new interests for our students. Psychologically, they derived a sense of accomplishment and, as a result, perhaps the ambition to tackle new challenges in the future. Colin particularly enjoyed it, volunteering time on weekends and staying after school to boil syrup. Students also learned the value of renewable forest resources, and they now know that not all syrups come from the grocery store shelf, chock full of corn syrup and preservatives! Furthermore, projects such as these build community among the staff, who work together instead of independently, as with the traditional concept of segregated classrooms.

For those schools on a limited budget, EE does not have to be expensive. During maple-tapping season, miniature syruping operations can be constructed outside or boiling can be done in incremental amounts over a stove (read about this first!) or an outdoor fire pit. The National Gardening Association provides grants to schools across the country to start school gardens. Another alternative is a "traveling box," a new, inexpensive tool for educators.[16] Teachers can order the self-contained, portable box from local natural resource agency offices or educational facilities for periods of a few days to a month. These boxes contain objects and materials on an environmental topic and can be incorporated into a variety of subjects. Studies have concluded that classes who used such materials show significant changes in knowledge. Students learn to understand human values and attitudes, as well as how to consider a range of practical solutions to the various assigned topics. The boxes also provide an alternative for teachers who lack the time required to prepare an extensive environmental program.

Many organizations, such as the National Gardening Association (see Appendix A for contact information), give grants to schools, and garden centers often will donate leftovers at the end of the year. Cooperative extensions at universities may provide someone certified as a "master gardener" to assist educators in preparing a garden.

One of the most effective interventions is to involve an ADHD student in tasks utilizing movement, although only 15 percent of respondents in one survey employed this intervention.[17] Specific rules and such expectations as sitting at a desk for long periods of time; not moving, making noise, or touching things; doing repetitive tasks; and encouraging compliance over creativity frustrate students with ADHD. Exercise strengthens the basal ganglia, the cerebellum, and the corpus callosum, facilitating neural connections.[18] Behavioral modification systems, such as token economies, class rules, and positive reinforcement, are effective, but the clinical picture of these adolescents tends to include restlessness. Exercise does not have to be limited to mundane activities but can be broadened to include hiking, biking, canoeing or kayaking, yoga, gardening, farming, or building, as further elaborated on in later chapters. Also, it is suggested to avoid unstructured settings, such as recess, and instead provide a structured physical activity in its place.

Environmental education is a possible intervention that would provide movement-oriented tasks. Perhaps the activity involved may stimulate dopamine, release of endorphins, the reticular activating system, and blood flow in the frontal lobes of the brain. Such tasks would also increase activity in the areas of the brain responsible for movement, located in the cerebral cortex. This activity was first discovered in 1864 by the German physicians Eduard Hitzig and Gustav Fritsch, who stimulated the cortical surface on living dogs and observed muscular contractions on the opposite sides of the body. Neuroscientists are seeking an actual neural link between areas in the brain involved with movement and those related to cognitive activity. The basal ganglia and the cerebellum are associated with the control of muscle movement, but these two areas are also important in coordinating thought processes. They are also connected to the frontal lobe area where planning the order and timing of future behavior occurs.[19] Thus, stimulating these areas through movement might facilitate one's ability to plan and consider consequences.

Actions are necessary to anchor thought, even an action such as talking. Talking stimulates the neurotransmitter acetylcholine. During talking, acetylcholine is released across synapses of activated neurons to stimulate muscle function. In turn, this stimulates dendritic growth and thus increases the network of neurons.[20] This is one reason why the lecture format often fails for many students, who sit quietly comatose in their seats because they have frequently been reprimanded for talking. The key component for these students is hands-on activity that actively, not passively, engages the brain. Infusing EE into general educational curricula as an "action learning" approach may be an effective intervention, addressing cognitive and social deficits in children with ADHD, in addition to a strengths assessment approach. Therefore, children, as well as adults, with ADHD may benefit from "experiential" learning as opposed to passive learning. However, many traditional and alternative educational curricula fail to incorporate an approach to learning that involves activity.

Author Laura Sewall states that ADHD is a decent alternative to simply going numb. Adolescents today are cramped in classrooms of thirty-five or more children, hear incessant bells, sit under artificial lighting, and listen to lectures that are most likely irrelevant to contemporary issues. "In other words, ADD represents a constellation of responses to a world that doesn't fit the true human condition . . . I mean the hunger for relevance, the desire of the body to move, to be of use, and, as a child, to play."[21]

David Orr stated in a 1990 commencement address to Arkansas College:

> Courses taught as lecture courses tend to induce passivity. Indoor classes create the illusion that learning only occurs inside four walls isolated from what students call without apparent irony the "real world." Dissecting frogs in biology classes teaches lessons about nature that no one would verbally profess. Campus architecture is crystallized pedagogy that often reinforces passivity, monologue, domination and artificiality.[22]

Students taught under these conditions may collectively experience a form of entropy as based on the second law of thermodynamics, the law of the dissipation of energy, formulated by the French physicist Sadi Carnot. Any isolated or "closed" physical system will proceed spontaneously in the direction of ever-increasing disorder; thus, entropy may be seen as a measure of disorder.[23]

Researchers analyzed data from the Longitudinal Study of American Youth (LSAY) and found that when students learn new information in meaningful contexts (under problem-solving conditions), they begin to understand the various circumstances in which to apply concepts and facts. The research indicated that young people are concerned about environmental issues, and, hence, teachers have an opportunity to use students' concerns as a source of motivation.[24]

Furthermore, instructional techniques that provide a purposeful, problem-oriented context for learning are more likely to prevent inert knowledge problems than techniques that employ a fact-oriented approach. The Cognition and Technology Group at Vanderbilt, in 1990, defined inert knowledge as knowledge that is not spontaneously used in problem solving but can be recalled when requested. The interdisciplinary nature of environmental problems provides an ideal opportunity for meaningful, integrated, and problem-oriented instruction.[25]

Certain states obviously are aware of the positive effects of EE. In 1990, Wisconsin legislature passed Act 299, requiring the periodic assessment of environmental literacy of Wisconsin's teachers and students.[26] The school code of the state of Illinois requires that environmental issues be discussed in the classroom. Teachers agreed that students should be guided in developing a set of values and feelings of concern for the environment, and that EE should be considered a priority in their K-12 school system. One major impediment is that few attempts have been made to involve teachers in developing a child's capacity for better problem-solving techniques in the classroom. [27] However, there are no national standards for environmental education; Pennsylvania is the only state that has separate standards.

Perhaps one model to emulate is that seen in Ontario Province in Canada, which has thirteen goals for public education. Two of these goals specify developing values related to personal, ethical, or religious beliefs; a respect for the environment; and a commitment to the wise use of resources. Thus, this supports the premise for environmental education in general education. The Ontario public education system has incorporated environmental education into the daily classroom routine; teachers are permitted to take their classes to special sites, and some boards of education have provided an environmental education program at a special field school.[28]

It is imperative that we advocate for the need to change traditional educational curricula, as well as traditional approaches to psychotherapy. Alternative solutions need to be proposed and implemented. In his book *Ecological Literacy, Education and the Transition to a Postmodern World,* Orr defines "ecological sustainability" as the task of finding alternatives to the practices that got us into trouble in the first place. He suggests it is necessary to rethink agriculture, shelter, energy use, urban design, transportation, economics, community patterns, resource use, forestry, the importance of wilderness, and our central values. This definition must also include education or "educational sustainability."

Sustainability is complex. It has been defined as the ability of a society to meet its needs without jeopardizing future generations or nonrenewable resources. "Uphold," "maintain," and "continue" are all synonyms for "sustain." Perhaps this also means that we should continue traditions from previous generations, but instead as technology advances, we are *rejecting* traditions and replacing them with anything that satisfies our immediate needs, whether those needs are convenient foods, machinery that creates pollution, or cramped classrooms. We need to find sustainable alternatives when traditional education and psychology cannot meet the needs of today's youths. Sustainability includes teaching others about maintaining those traditions which are desirable and viable from one generation to the next. This implies a responsibility to instill values in students, which can be accomplished through education and community service, or can simply begin at home. If one's self-image changes because of community, as based on Margaret Mead's theory mentioned in the preface, then perhaps virtues of sustainability may be taught in the context of a community. Certainly, sustainability may be taught through tapping maple trees and boiling syrup with students. Camping excursions may also teach one about renewable forest resources, and farming enhances one's connections with the earth and appreciation of the food given to us by the earth.

Should we continue to teach using traditional methods because alternatives are too time-consuming? Should we continue to churn out high school and college graduates who are ill equipped and inadequately prepared for the rest of their lives? Aside from integrating environmental education into curricula and therapy, we need to revive the trade industry, including woodworking and carpentry. These are not defunct professions, and if we continue to concentrate our focus on technology and investment banking, we will suffer the loss of skilled laborers.

We often misinterpret behavior, attributing it to the individual and not the environment. A passive classroom learning environment is going to induce restlessness in one with hyperactivity, one who needs to be engaged in experiential tasks. As I have stated earlier and cannot emphasize enough, we need to implement changes in the external system, not necessarily alter the individual through medication and short-term therapy. Vocational schools do satisfy a need for experiential training, but students who are slotted for the standard college preparatory courses do not qualify. What happens if students are interested in farming and gardening with the intention of teaching someday or becoming naturalists? Do they have to spend years searching for another career path? Hopefully, they stumble into other people who will encourage such interests, but do we want to rely on coincidence? Orr writes that students today are occupied with subtracting, multiplying, dividing, and computing. However, it is essential that we have farmers, foresters, writers, and businesspersons who are ecologically literate and can build the foundation for sustainable solutions.[29]

It seems apparent that those with learning disabilities do not design educational curricula. As Orr states, conferences in expensive settings exclude people with calloused hands.[30] One of the conceits of modern science is the belief that it can be applied everywhere in the same manner. Global exchange economy treats all parts of the world the same regardless of varying ecological conditions. And so, this appears to be the case for education and psychology.

In *The Unsettling of America,* Wendell Berry expresses frustration with present-day "practical education," as opposed to liberal education:

> One studies the *Divine Comedy* and the Pythagorean theorem not to acquire something to be exchanged for something else, but to understand the orders and the kinds of thought and to furnish the mind with subjects and examples. Because the standards are rooted in examples, they do not change.[31]

Berry laments that today's "practical education" is oriented to the future and is left to the whim of instructors who define the future, believing that students need to be equipped with skills that will enable them to make money.

Today, practicality is synonymous with money, whereas once upon a time, practicality was associated with a particular lifestyle, such as farming or other earth-sustaining activities. Practicality today does not include ecologically based programs that focus on gardening, farming, and forest and land preservation. "Practical" careers that guarantee high incomes include computer programming, Web design, and banking. Students are taught that the underlying emphasis and focus in life is money. Who cares if we destroy 150 square miles of forest every day? As long as we have the biggest sport utility vehicle (SUV) and "McMansion" on the block, what else do we need? I am merely regurgitating what I hear from many of today's adolescents. This ensures employment for many psychologists, who benefit in the long run, listening to their bored, wealthy clients complain of "communication gaps" with their spouses who spend exorbitant amounts of time at work to pay mortgages and credit card debts.

Happiness has become a lost attribute, as children are shuffled from sport to sport, program to program, and fed "time-saving" frozen dinners without ever once questioning their origin, other than the freezer. Is it any wonder that several million doses of Prozac are administered daily in the United States?

Social work focuses on person-in-the-environment, but "environment" is not limited to just social factors. One must take into account the physical, cultural, and natural surroundings and how these factors simultaneously interact to influence behavior. Behavior and the environment are an interactive system. Behavior changes when the environmental stimuli change. Conversely, we can change behavior by changing the relevant stimuli.

Kurt Lewin's field theory states that the person and the person's environment operate together in an integral way within the immediate "field of time." At any given time, behavior *(B)* is a function *(f)* of the person *(P)* and the environment *(E)*:

$$B = f(P + E)$$

Behavior *(B)*, as defined by Lewin, is a product of the combination of environmental and psychological factors. The person *(P)* encompasses all psychological, internal events, including dreaming, thinking, and acting. Environmental factors *(E)* refer to the immediate, external interaction with other people and can be divided into the physical environment and the social environment. Physical environment is defined as time and place, whereas the social environment is the implied presence or participation of others. According to this theory, behavior is the direct result of both the individual and the environment. The one limitation to this theory is that it focuses on immediate time and neglects the role of historic causation.[32]

The theory of planned behavior accounts for historic causation. It is based on the theory of reasoned action, that humans are rational beings who make systematic use of information available to them.[33]

Based on one's life experiences and the confidence that results from these experiences, one is more likely to perform certain behaviors.

Life span developmental theory seeks to explain behavioral responses as a consequence of life events. Life span development is multidimensional, including social, biological, and psychological dimensions.[34] This theory suggests that the influence of life events must be included as a central explanatory factor in behavioral analysis. Thus, if environmental education has positive effects, such as maintaining attention, increasing self-esteem and knowledge, and identifying new vocational interests, then it can be referred to as a life event that influences behavior, including the symptoms of ADHD. Ecological literacy teaches students to ask, "What then?" It implies the ability to think broadly, beyond conventional categories.[35] Biophilia, the affinity for the living world, begins in childhood, driven by a sense of wonder, the sheer delight in being alive in this beautiful, mysterious world.

However, there are innumerable impediments to overcome. The unfortunate reality is that environmental education is taught approximately only half an hour per week on a nationwide level. Education has evolved into an indoor activity. David Orr concludes that environmental education is still superfluous and will be disregarded during budget restrictions and that our educational institutions do not address the issues raised by the challenge of sustainability. And if they are represented in agricultural colleges and schools supported by the Education Land Grant Act, then ecology and environmental programs are still segregated. I discovered environmental education by accident because I happened to live on the agricultural campus during graduate school. What if environmental education had been instilled in me at a young age? I always worshipped nature, but not once did I ever hear of farming or environmental education throughout my years of torturous traditional education.

Orr argues that issues of environment and those of sustainability are complex and long-term, while politics addresses more immediate issues such as jobs and crime. Politicians who talk about complex issues and difficult choices presumably do not win elections. This can be generalized to anyone attempting to implement change, as is evident in Pennsylvania, where I now live and work. It is disheartening and saddening to see applications for charter schools, particularly environmental charter schools, denied.

On a microlevel, it is relatively easy to build a community garden in a school. However, on a macrolevel, when one wants to start a new school, introduce a different curriculum, and employ teachers who deviate from established tradition, one can anticipate many obstacles and hurdles to overcome. Is it a case of ignorance is bliss? Does this call for education and learning on the part of our administrators, comfortable in their air-conditioned offices and with their uncalloused hands? Does it demand an increase in work hours? Maybe it is possible to teach an old dog new tricks, but maybe the dog *does not want to learn*.

This resistance to change our educational system is similar to the principle of "least cost" choices. Orr notes that economically, rational, self-interested people will know that least cost is not always the same as true cost. Food prices do not include the cost of topsoil, groundwater depletion or contamination, stream destruction, health care for farmers and farm workers, or subsidies for public water in the West. If we paid the true costs of production, prices would be considerably higher, as reflected in organic food. Are we adopting a "least cost" philosophy for education?

*   *   *

I have just finished a morning of teaching as a guest artist at the 1860 House, an old farm in Skillman, New Jersey, that integrates the teaching of art and environmental education. Local artists in the community exhibit in the gallery, as well as teach to community children ranging from five to twelve years old. Catherine Vaucher is the energetic director, coordinating the year-round program that provides outreach programs to inner-city youths as well as programs specifically for learning-disabled students. As I have previously mentioned, the wonders of the environment and teaching these wonders never cease to amaze me.

I led the same hike three times this morning for three different age groups, even though I was somewhat cranky from lack of sleep and humid temperatures soaring into the high nineties. The theme this week is wildlife and that is the only mandate I have to follow. This morning, we investigated animal tracks and made nature journals. I told them we were going to be "naturalists" today. The most succinct definition for a five-year-old that I can offer is "one who loves and studies nature and teaches others." They seemed to grasp it.

Accustomed to teaching high school adolescents, I was initially a bit wary working with young children again. However, once on the trail, their enthusiasm and wide-eyed wonder was infectious and I was granted the opportunity to see nature through their eyes, something I need to nurture in myself. At these times I am fully absorbed in the moment. Clutching their nature journals and pencils, they gleefully shouted, "Look—a deer track!" Everyone raced over, hunched over their books, and, with all the manual dexterity five-year-olds can muster, attempted to draw a "V." It was precious and touching to see. I cannot ever believe that I once despised children!

The group continued along the trail, and I was surprised at their excitement, always fresh, always new. Yet another deer track elicited cries of excitement from them, and again when they spotted the exoskeleton of a cicada. In fact, one girl picked it up and curiously examined it, to my delight. Although I had to repeat the class twice more with varying age groups, every group brought my attention to something I had previously bypassed. A year ago, I probably would have quit after the first day, bored by the repetition. However, we always discovered a new track, be it that of a raccoon, deer, or cottontail rabbit. They consistently provided me with a new perspective, seeing things I did not. We think we teach children, yet they teach us much about life.

Friends and family have opened my eyes as well. I lived on a canal for a year and sometimes tired of biking on it. However, one evening I biked with my friends Margaret and Mike, who pointed out creatures I'd not seen before on the canal: a swimming beaver, a large turtle, and a beautiful blue heron. From then on, I attempted to see something new each time I biked on the canal, whether a tree I'd not identified or some creature. I had the opportunity last spring to watch the ducks perform their mating rituals and, consequently, rear their offspring.

Although this chapter has focused on incorporating EE into schools as an experiential therapy for adolescents with ADD/ADHD, EE is also proposed as alternative therapy for adults with ADD/ADHD. Ecopsychology programs introduce groups to hiking and camping, for example, and integrate journal writing to allow participants to express and link emotions to nature. For some, these experiences may encourage the expression of repressed emotions and result in similar psychological and social benefits similar to the effects of EE on children, as discussed earlier in this chapter.

B. F. Skinner wrote, "The individualist can find no solace in reflecting upon any contribution which will survive him. He has refused to act for the good of others and is therefore not reinforced by the fact that others whom he has helped will outlive him. He has refused to be concerned for the survival of his culture and is not reinforced by the fact that the culture will long survive him."[36] The inference is that evolution selects cultures that do manage to get people to care about the next generation.[37]

We may never understand the consequences of our actions while we are living, but a sense of morality should engender our behavior. As Wendell Berry writes:

> To use knowledge and tools in a particular place with good long-term results is not heroic. It is not a grand action visible for a long distance or a long time. It is a small action, but more complex and difficult, more skillful and responsible, more whole and enduring, than most grand actions. It comes of a willingness to devote oneself to work that perhaps only the eye of Heaven will see in its full intricacy and excellence. Perhaps the real work, like real prayer and real charity, must be done in secret.[38]

With the close of this chapter, I ask the reader to consider the statistics that follow as yet one more reason why environmental education should be incorporated into every educational curriculum in the country.

- Fifteen thousand to 20,000 people die annually from respiratory conditions directly related to air quality; most are minorities and the poor.
- One percent of global warming comes from Los Angeles alone.
- Some scientists predict that by the middle of this century, global warming will result in most of the coastal cities in the United States being below sea level.
- Each hour, five square miles of the rainforest are destroyed; by the end of the year, this area of destruction will be the size of Pennsylvania.
- Air pollution has created a hole in the ozone layer as big as the United States.

- Acid rain, besides destroying the lakes and forests, is now considered to be the leading cause of lung cancer after cigarette smoke.
- Thirty-five thousand people die from starvation every day.
- Two or more species become extinct every day due to deforestation and pollution.
- Farmland harvest area per person has decreased to half of what it was in 1950 because we have converted farmland to residential use.
- Topsoil losses equal approximately 7 percent each decade, and result from wind and water erosion emptying into streams, lakes, and oceans.
- It is projected that we will run out of usable water within the next thirty years; rainwater can no longer replenish aquifers because deforestation, urbanization, and overgrazing increase run-off.
- Sixty percent of people living in rural areas of third-world countries do not have safe drinking water.
- Less than one-third of the world's original forest still remains, and the United States has only 5 percent left; in 1994, only 5 percent of the world's lumber was grown sustainably.
- Carbon emissions are the highest in 160,000 years, increasing exponentially since the sixteenth century.
- Since 1880, the earth's temperature has risen about one degree Fahrenheit; only a few degrees more will decrease farmland production, force agriculture toward the poles, and require new dams, irrigation, and migration of human populations.
- Measurable amounts of mercury, DDT, industrial chemicals, plastic, oil, and sewage sludge have been detected in our oceans at sites previously thought to be pollution free.

Chapter 4

Reaping What You Sow

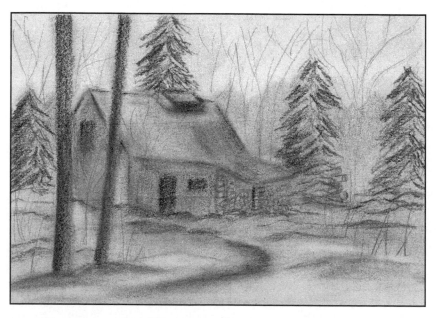

The seed on good soil stands for those with a noble and good heart, who hear the word, retain it, and by persevering, produce a good crop.

Luke 8:15

After my internship at Stony Brook ends, my friend Scott invites me to work with him on an organic farm in New Hampshire. The first day I arrive we pull 2,500 onions, thin beets, and harvest Brandywine tomatoes, trying to beat the ominous threat of rain. I find myself in the barn snipping onions at midnight for the farmer's market at six the next morning. Andre, the farmer, leases 200 acres situated on rolling green pastures surrounded by dense foliage. One morning I rise before those faint tinges of pink streak the sky and walk a mile up the narrow, gravel drive to midmeadow. Here tall sunflowers dance in the morning breeze, their heads swaying to a faint rhythm only they can hear. Sometimes after midnight when a full moon illuminates the fields, I sit in the open meadow and stargaze at the clear New England sky, a pinhole shade of eternal dots of light. The katydids, crickets, and cicadas serenade me, a beautiful, ethereal chorus.

On earth, however, the septic system has completely broken down prior to my arrival, leaving us without any plumbing. A shovel and toilet paper appear on the steps outside. It is a chaotic few days, as Andre stays up for the duration of each night, laying pipe for a new system. Once it is fixed, life on the farm resumes—essentially we work fewer hours.

During my visit, I have the opportunity to work a farmer's market in Hampton with Scott. We drive to the Hampton market and set up a portable farm stand, a conglomeration of wooden boards and a large white canopy, in the parking lot. Other farmers pull up in pickups, quickly setting up in a similar manner. We arrange the vegetables and bunches of dried flowers in baskets. Soon, the parking lot is bustling with customers, and money changes hands in exchange for a multitude of fresh, organic produce. I help weigh produce and collect money.

The farm stand across from us attracts my eye, and I go over and talk to the Asian woman behind it. She is from Thailand and tells me about the mycology farm she and her husband own in Stratham. They grow shiitake mushrooms, an incredibly tasty and "meaty" mushroom that grows on the shii tree, a type of beech tree. She eagerly shows me a book depicting pictures of the growth stages and explains that shiitake mushrooms grow during the hotter months of July and August when temperatures are in the eighties on a daily basis. They do not appear difficult to grow, and I add this to the list inside my head for future reference! I sample a mushroom and finish helping with the farm stand. Other farmers sell similar produce, baked goods, such as fresh bread and homemade granola, and feta cheese. The time passes quickly, and I feel a sense of pride, selling this food, knowing I have helped to harvest it and it will be part of someone's meal tonight.

The following spring, I journey once again to New Hampshire to work with Scott for a long weekend on a 500-acre maple sugar farm near Mount Kearsarge. I arrive after dark, following the long, twisty gravel road up the mountain and through the woods. Just as I think my car cannot endure one more pothole, my high beams illuminate the last driveway. I get out and stretch my muscles, cramped after the six-hour drive. A swinging lantern emits rays through the darkness, and Scott's face appears, the light displacing shadows on his face in an eerie manner. I hug him tightly. His determination to pursue a farming career is remarkable and admirable. Indeed, he is one of the most remarkable people I know.

He leads the way inside and introduces me to Jennifer and Bob, who appear to be in their midforties, the owners, and husband and wife. Bob is quite a character. A long entangled beard conceals much of his face; a hat perches atop his wild hair. He smiles broadly, revealing a missing side tooth, and his eyes crinkle into deep creases when he smiles. Jennifer is petite and sports a blunt haircut. I admire her forearms, lean and veined from logging. She proudly describes cutting trees during her eighth month of pregnancy.

Bob bought the land sixteen years ago, pitching a tent while he built the house in which he, Jennifer, and his two children presently live. He and Jennifer log, raise sheep, tap maple sugar trees in the spring, and organically farm vegetables and hay. Their house is constructed from beautiful hemlock and pine and is a work in progress, with plans to extend the master bedroom and kitchen. A generator supplies them with electricity and the lamps are battery powered. I am entranced with the stove built in the 1940s, which is fueled by wood, generating enough heat for the house. I am awed and inspired by their lifestyle.

Exhausted, sleep overcomes me, and due to space restrictions, we camp out in sleeping bags in an unfinished room. Scott stokes the woodstove and its warmth fills the room, despite outside temperatures in the thirties. I read him one of my favorite Wendell Berry poems, "To Know the Dark," and "I Saw in Louisiana a Live Oak Growing" by Walt Whitman, as the light of the nearby lantern flickers on the pages. He reads "Meditation in the Spring Rain," also by Berry, and I am lulled into a peaceful slumber.

The bleating of bloated ewes awakens us in the wee hours of dawn. Jennifer excitedly tells me they are expecting a birth any day. After breakfast, we venture out to the barn and stables, where eighteen sheep and two horses reside. No baby lamb yet. Scott doles out their food and then we wander down to the sap house. The sap house, constructed of tin and aluminum, overlooks a nearby pond and distant mountains. Unfortunately, due to unseasonably warm weather, the sap has ceased its run. Alternating days of warmth and freezing nights are necessary catalysts for the sap to run. Once the trees sense a certain warmth, their buds begin to swell and the taste is corrupted. Instead, we prepare to close the sap house, cleaning out the boiler pan, vigorously scrubbing the sides, and hoisting the smokestack up through the roof. We help Bob fill the remaining jugs of syrup and Scott explains the tapping process to me. Buckets collect sap from the taps in nearby trees, but on extensive property, pipes are run from tree to tree where the sap drains into 300-gallon tubs scattered throughout their property and is later pumped into the sap house. It is then funneled into the boiler pan, heated to 7.1 to 7.5 degrees Fahrenheit above the boiling point of water, transferred to the finishing pan, and drained into jugs to go to farm markets and stores. Syrup is sold in different grades, ranging from A to C, or utility syrup. Bob wrinkles his nose at utility syrup, explaining that is the heaviest, darkest, most molasseslike syrup. Within each grade, there are colors: light, medium, and dark amber. Light, or fancy, is the ultimate syrup.

During the afternoon, I take a break and meander down the brook to Bob's teepee supported with maple sugar tree trunks and canvas. I peek inside. Two futons and a fire pit furnish the area. Scott tells me Bob lives out there in the summertime, listening to Red Sox games on his radio under the stars. I snicker and comment on it as a fantastic survival tactic for marriage. Bob seems amused.

Scott and I break shortly before sunset and hike around the property, taking pictures. We examine tree trunks and leaves, admiring the brilliant white birches, hemlocks, sugar maples, and beeches. He points out the difference between sugar and Norway maple leaves, the former having smooth lobe edges and the latter with dentate, or toothed, edges. We hike to a part of the forest where the trees no longer bear leaves, their branches stark and barren due to beaver damage. It is a graveyard, reminding me of the finite nature of life. We travel on, hopping across brooks, and sit by a beautiful frozen waterfall at sunset, watching the water cascade over the rocks in the creek bed. It is breathtakingly beautiful. We walk back to the house to help prepare a vegetable lasagna and salad and settle in for the evening, reading and falling asleep to John Coltrane's crooning saxophone.

The next morning, a surprise greets us: twin baby lambs! Scott attempts to hold them for a picture, but the mother steadfastly refuses. I settle for a picture from the fence. After admiring the newborns for a while, it is time to begin the day's work. We clean over 200 sap buckets, drenched in water and wading in sheep manure, while Bob bulldozes the largest compost pile I have ever seen. I cherish the warm shower later, and that night, we drive to a neighbor's house for a poetry and art gathering. Bob serenades us with folk songs, launching into a great rendition of "Uncle John's Band." Scott insists I bring my art portfolio, consisting of color photographs of my paintings. Hesitantly, I agree. Once a month, old friends gather to swap talk of politics, poetry, and art. Scott reads Wendell Berry's poem, "Contrariness of the Mad Farmer," which I wholeheartedly embrace, enjoying Berry's inherent rebellious nature. I reluctantly pass around my portfolio. To my surprise, people comment quite positively, which elicits a smile from me. Ah, I thought. This is what the gift of creativity is about, not keeping it to one's self. It is to share and inspire, and that is the greatest enjoyment I derive from my art.

It is a wonderful group of people, comprised of a local potter, an artist, and farmers. I amusedly watch one woman throughout the evening, intently drawing the man sitting next to her. She rarely glances up, participating very sporadically in the conversation. I almost feel the pencil in my hand, how akin I have become to drawing once again. The evening evolves into talk of farming politics and the plight of small-scale organic farming, the worries and demands. The hard life is reflected in their weathered faces. At the end of the evening, we drive home and collapse into bed. I depart the next morning, and I am, as always, brokenhearted to leave New England.

However, an inner tranquility eases my spirits. Once home, I resume my studies at the Fleisher Art Memorial in Philadelphia, a tuition-free art school established by the late multimillionaire Samuel Fleisher. It is a still-life class and, feeling very whimsical, I paint a quite abstract still life of a vase, violin case, and bowl in vibrant oranges, reds, and blues. My teacher comments on what an "interesting, strange piece." I am pleased with it and attribute this release of creativity to my farming adventures.

Farming interests me greatly. I enjoy the manual, physical labor and lifestyle and include as much organic food in my diet as possible. I work sporadically on organic farms and savor every bite of Brandywine tomatoes, fresh raw corn-on-the-cob, succulent eight ball zucchini, jalapeno peppers, tomatillos, and baby bell peppers. Wild edible plants such as milkweed, ramps, and asparagus fill my palate.

*   *   *

Why farming for ADD? First, it involves constant physical and manual labor. As previously mentioned, movement boosts serotonin levels, a deficiency found in those with ADD/ADHD. Unlike traditional study, with farming I do not feel lethargic; I am alert and enthusiastic about what I am learning and the tasks sustain my attention. I am willing to go so far as to suggest that there may be a link between farming and the reticular activating system.

Second, it is visual learning. Reading supplements my limited knowledge of farming, but I understand concepts such as soil composition and nutrient cycles when I see it for myself, as do many of my students. For instance, we pack jars of soil from our school garden and allow the layers to stratify into sand, silt, and clay. How many of them would comprehend this explanation from reading a textbook in a classroom versus actually seeing it in an experiment from our garden? We also use soil test kits to determine the pH, phosphorous, potassium, and nitrogen levels from soil samples. I split them into groups, and they eagerly fill the tubes, anxiously waiting for the results.

One summer, my co-worker Stephanie and I worked with four girls from a foster home designing and building a farm stand to sell our produce. As a group, we initially designed it on paper, integrating geometric formulas such as the Pythagorean theorem. Although geometry is typically taught indoors, it can be taught on an interactive level and experientially in such woodworking and carpentry projects. EE also involves other mathematical concepts: measurement, weights, graphing, recording data, designing, and observational skills. The students work together to formulate a solution instead of struggling alone with pencil and paper. Students working as a group toward a tangible goal generates enthusiasm. In addition, I have observed students directly give one another support, encouragement, and praise during these group endeavors. Students also conquer fears of learning; one student admitted a fear of math and refused to measure a piece of wood. We worked with her to read the tape measure, and she triumphantly smiled when she measured a piece on her own, her eyes aglow with pride.

Third, farming builds community and group cohesion, as well as providing the many psychological and social benefits mentioned in the previous chapter. Students readily help one another and staff members. Such cooperation lends a sense of accomplishment as, together, we cook and eat food fresh from our garden, providing lessons in nutrition.

Fourth, there is an interminable amount to learn about farming, such as plant physiology, botany, seed structure, fruits, vegetables, and soil chemistry. Opening one book leads to another and yet another.

Fifth, farming is one positive way to channel addictive behaviors, anger, and depression. If movement does indeed boost serotonin and one is so engaged in the work, learning new concepts and immersed in a world of radiant beauty, then this may be one likely antidote for depression and addiction. It is a natural high that far surpasses a chemical high. If farming ignites the hunger for knowledge in someone, an insatiable craving to acquire knowledge may develop. Hangovers are banished to the past; they consume too much energy and are a frivolous waste of precious time that may be spent outside harvesting vegetables, tilling the land, or hiking in the forest and inhaling the scent of white pines. Farming is a cognitive-behavioral form of therapy for drug and alcohol addiction, as studies have found that exercise is more effective than traditional psychotherapy in alleviating drug and alcohol problems. People with drug and alcohol problems in traditional psychotherapy programs reported higher rates of relapses.[1]

Farming may also be considered a cognitive or rational-emotive form of therapy, as maladaptive thought processes may be restructured; one is challenged on a daily basis. Learning concepts such as soil science may increase self-esteem as one acquires knowledge and gains confidence in one's abilities, thus enhancing self-efficacy. If one can learn to grow one's own food, is that not enhancing self-efficacy? Perhaps one decides to pursue a career as a farmer, horticulturalist, plant geneticist, or biologist. Furthermore, these are tangible results as opposed to traditional psychotherapy's emphasis on cognitive results. Positive thoughts replace the downward spiral of negative thoughts that one often feels trapped in and experiences, an overwhelming sensation of drowning with no hope of resurfacing.

Sixth, maintaining an organic food diet improves health and provides energy, as explained further in this chapter. By enhancing one's diet, often a benefit of farming and gardening, health invariably improves. In one study, DHA, an omega-3 fatty acid (as discussed later in this chapter), increased P300 waves (see Chapter 1), which are often decreased in those with ADD/ADHD.

Farming may reap the same benefits as meditation, teaching one patience and the ability to focus on a task, thus keeping one from distracting thoughts. Farming, as a meditative activity, may induce alpha waves, another possible deficit in those with ADD/ADHD. Farming also teaches mindfulness, as it creates a full awareness of living in the present moment. This results in an increase in one's patience, and I have personally found it to be a technique for anger management, an outlet for channeling aggression and frustration. Farming has taught me great patience in daily life, including in my interactions with others. Living on a farm has irrevocably changed my life; it is a drastic reduction in the frenetic pace at which most people live. Because I am not bombarded by extraneous stimuli, the silence allows me to deeply contemplate my thoughts. It is appalling now to drive on the highway when I visit friends and family in other states, outside country life. People speed recklessly by, honk horns, and shout expletives. Parking lots are accidents waiting to happen and, as a result, tempers flare left and right. It is suddenly so apparent what an angry and rude society we live in, a society based on convenience and productivity. The congestion, noise, and pollution are enough to provoke a nervous breakdown in any healthy person. My greatest days are watching a cow meander in the road, holding up "traffic," perhaps a car or two. As the sun sets, I take lengthy bike rides past neighboring farms, inhaling the pungent scent of cow manure, and watch baby lambs frolic in the pastures.

Finally, it is the lifestyle that appeals to me the most. Farming demands excessive energy for the arduous, physical labor, yet paradoxically it is relaxing. It is a return to an agrarian past. I spend very little time in my car these days. Hands down, I'd choose picking blueberries any day over sitting in a traffic jam, inhaling carbon monoxide fumes. Cooking and eating butternut squash soup made from your own produce in the company of friends is an ideal way to spend fall and winter evenings. I find great enjoyment picking fresh arugula and radishes from my garden for a spring salad. Farm markets are an opportunity

to swap stories, produce, and advice and to build friendships with local farmers.

Berry writes:

> We lose our health—and create profitable diseases and
> dependences—by failing to see the direct connections between
> living and eating, eating and working, working and loving. In
> gardening, for instance, one works with the body to feed the
> body. The work, if it is knowledgeable, makes for excellent
> food. And it makes one hungry. The work thus makes eating
> both nourishing and joyful, not consumptive, and keeps the
> eater from getting fat and weak. This is health, wholeness, a
> source of delight.[2]

* * *

It is not long before I return to New Hampshire in August. After a
frenetic week of teaching environmental education and painting at
the 1860 House, I dash up to Andre's one Friday afternoon in mid-
August. How many people who are burned out after working all summer drive six hours and volunteer to work on a farm? Sometimes I
think I need to have my head examined . . . or so I've been told.

I arrive late Friday night after battling construction traffic in Hart-
ford. My heart leaps as I turn into the gravel driveway. I squeeze my
car into a parking space in the crowded driveway and jump out. I stretch
and inhale the fresh, clean New England air. The moon brightly illuminates my path. The farmhouse is ablaze in light, welcoming and inviting. I walk in and spot Hilary, Andre's housemate, sitting at a table
with some other people, talking and laughing. She is a wonderful person and is managing the farm stand across the street this summer.
Scott ventures into the kitchen and I throw my arms around him.

Three of Andre's friends have driven up from New Brunswick to
help out for the weekend. After a flurry of activity, some homemade
brewed beer supplied by one of Andre's friends, and conversation, we
do not get to sleep until two. Scott tells me we are getting up at four to
pick corn before market. I laugh and tell him to make up another joke.
He is not kidding. After teaching all morning and driving 350 miles, I
politely tell him to exclude the "we" from this conversation!

I settle in to sleep later and just as it seems I've drifted off to sleep,
my eyes flutter open. Doors are opening and closing, feet walking up

and down the stairs. The room is dark; moonlight filters onto the floorboards. The crickets and cicadas are chirping away in the surrounding fields. It cannot possibly be four, but it is. Fortunately, I get to sleep in. Andre tells me later that when he tried to wake me, I kept mumbling over and over, "It can't be four . . . it's not possible."

When I open my eyes again, the house is quiet. I peek out the window, trying to determine the time. Gray stratus clouds converge overhead. Feeling guilty for sleeping in, I lace up my boots, pull on some work pants and a tank top. Downstairs, the clock reads 8:30. I decide to hike up to midmeadow about a half mile away and see who is working there. Majestic shagbark hickories line the drive and a cool breeze rustles the leaves. When I reach midmeadow, I gaze in surprise. Fields of goldenrod, purple loosestrife, black-eyed Susans, chicory, and thistle run wild where an abundance of crops once grew. I then recall that Andre recently purchased farmland across the street and assume that is where he has planted new crops. I walk back to the house and spot a figure in the nearby meadow. Trudging through rampant weeds, I stop to admire planted wildflowers, rows of gladiolas, asters, snapdragons, blooming in vibrant hues of rose, crimson, violet, and maize. They are dried, bunched together, and sold at market.

I walk closer to the hunched-over figure, who is harvesting zucchini, squash, and peppers, the only remaining crops this side of the street. I recognize the woman under the hat as Sylvan, a friend of Andre's I met last year. Sylvan tells me she is working on a postdoctorate in ecology at Harvard. We rummage through rows and harvest bell peppers, eight ball zucchini, and yellow patty pan summer squash. We load her car and drive across the street to unload and distribute some to Andre's farm stand. The rest goes to the greenhouse to be washed and stored for farm markets in nearby towns. Scott pokes his head inside the greenhouse and asks me to help him harvest yet more zucchini, squash, and peppers in the newly planted fields. We haul several more bushels into the back of Scott's "new" 1988 Ranger pickup and drive them to the greenhouse. I help Sylvan wash tubs and tubs of vegetables, while Scott picks tomatoes in the greenhouse. Suddenly, he yells.

"Amy! Sylvan! Come quick!"

Thinking tomato plants have attacked him or the greenhouse ceiling is caving in, we rush over. The greenhouse is a jungle of tomato plants, thick with green foliage.

"Where are you?" we yell.

"On the left!" says a disembodied voice.

Gently parting the rows of tomato plants, we rush inside. Scott is intently staring at a plant.

"This is the first hornworm I've ever seen," he mutters, partly to us, partly to himself. The tomato hornworm is well camouflaged and resembles a massive green caterpillar, clinging to the vine. Small white horns actually protrude from its head. This worm, as with the aphid, is a detrimental pest that devours tomato plants. Scott extracts a pair of pliers from his pocket and squeezes it. I cringe and turn away. The others comment on the green tomato plant juice oozing from its intestines.

Scott asks Sylvan and me if we would pick blueberries while he takes a nap. I relent as I have slept a couple more hours. We collect buckets from the farm stand and meander out to the blueberry bushes. There are about ten rows of blueberry bushes, and we happily gorge ourselves "taste testing" tart and sweet berries. It takes a good hour to fill our buckets halfway, but the time passes quickly as we swap teaching experiences and share our disdain for lecture format teaching, both of us preferring interactive learning. I reminisce about picking raspberries in Iowa on my great-uncle's 200-acre farm. Suddenly, Sylvan decides we have picked enough blueberries and should make blueberry pancakes—right now. Sounds great to me, so we head back to the farm stand, leave the blueberries with Hilary, and return to the house with a pint of blueberries for pancakes. We rummage through cookbooks, find a recipe, and mix up a batch. Scott wanders in, bleary-eyed from his nap, and wolfs down some pancakes. It is now my turn to succumb to sleep and I nap for a good hour.

At five, I wake and suddenly remember I need to make a couscous salad for the potluck supper. Andre is amused at my lack of planning, as I need chickpeas, which need to soak overnight. A minor modification, but I scrap the recipe for a basil, tomato, and fresh mozzarella couscous salad, and substitute Vermont cheddar cheese in lieu of the fresh mozzarella. Somehow, the couscous salad is assembled and people filter in. Bob and Jennifer drive down from Warner, and I am excited to show them the painting of their sap house I recently completed as part of a new series on farming.

Bob and Jennifer seem happily surprised with the sap house. Although it is a small canvas, I invested a considerable amount of time on it, using a wide brush with quick strokes and beautiful grays mixed from ultramarine blue and burnt sienna. I immersed myself in it, not setting deadlines and painting over it until I was satisfied. Unfortunately, productivity sometimes takes precedence over enjoyment. The evening is interesting, and I absorb myself in conversations on art and CSA (community-supported agriculture) farming. We also share dreams of owning a farm. However, by midnight, I walk outside and admire the beautiful luminescent moon. It is almost full and brilliantly illuminates the sky, masking the surrounding stars in a halo of light. The chill of the New England air wraps itself around my arms, hinting of fall. Serenity envelops me and, for a solipsistic moment, nothing exists but the moon and me. I do not move for a while, mesmerized by the stillness and magic of the night. Reluctantly, I tear myself away, ready to turn in for the evening.

The next morning, we are in the fields by 7:00 to pick corn. I have never picked corn and am excited at the prospect. I am not quite leaping out of bed, but getting out of it and being stimulated by the fresh morning air is a good start. The morning is cool and overcast, but nevertheless beautiful. Scott quickly moves down the rows, feeling the husks. With a quick, downward motion, he breaks off an ear.

"You want to feel for the rounded tops under the husks. Leave the pointed ones." He demonstrates and pulls back a husk, revealing a pointed top.

"See? No good . . . and look, an ear worm." He tosses it into a nearby field. He continues down the row and breaks off another ear, pulls off the outer husk, revealing a round top and yellow, glistening rows of corn.

"Want to do the honors?" he says and offers me the tantalizing corn. I nod and sink my teeth into the juicy corn. Perfect and sweet. He takes a bite, nods his approval and tosses it into the field.

"So, now, break off a stalk to use as a gate, to mark where you've started. Put the basket about forty feet in front of you and circle around. We'll only collect seven bushels today. We collected thirty-five yesterday."

Whew. I start eyeing the rows of corn, searching for an average size, feeling the tops. I am slow and awkward at first but eventually increase my speed. The corn tears easily once I learn the downward motion and establish a cyclic rhythm. It is gratifying and cathartic work. We haul the bushels into the back of the truck and drop them off at the farm stand.

Next, we drive out to the fields to harvest zucchini and squash. The leaves prick my fingers as I rummage through the rows, searching for zucchini and squash. I collect a bushel and then return to the greenhouse to wash and sort pickling and slicing cucumbers, zucchini, and yellow squash. We immerse them in large tubs of water and then quickly rub off dirt and place them in clean buckets. It amazes me that, although it is almost 11:30, I have amassed so much energy. Typically, I am still lethargic and feeling "foggy." All the activity stimulates me; I feel alert and highly focused.

It seems quite paradoxical that I can tolerate the repetition of farming tasks, such as cleaning vegetables or picking blueberries for an hour, or even two. Once upon a time, I would have quit after five minutes. Meditation has taught me much about patience and stillness. Farming is meditative; the patience it teaches you leads to the clarity of a greater picture.

Monday morning I clean beets in the greenhouse with Brandon, a new employee. It is pouring outside and about fifty-five degrees. I am drenched to the bone from picking blueberries and harvesting. The rain beats steadily on the plastic greenhouse ceiling.

"So do you want to farm someday?" I inquire.

"No way," he says, shaking his head. "Too boring. It's mindless."

"I used to feel exactly that way. It feels that way initially, but one day I realized that I had started to acquire and accumulate so much knowledge. Knowledge about the nutrient cycles of nitrogen, phosphorous and potassium deficiencies, diseased plants, edible plants, the growth and seasonal cycles of plants . . . and so much more. You can see each task as mundane or look at it as part of a larger picture. Each task is meditative . . . the more time I spend farming, the more I see how it is all integrated together. It teaches me to move with nature, to rise with the sun, sleep with the moon." I pause for a breath and hope I'm not rambling. I look at Brandon, hoping he has not fallen asleep, but he appears to be listening and slowly nods.

"Yeah, that makes sense."

"So, give it some time. You may change your mind as well." I plunge my hands back into the tub and continue washing beets, scrubbing dirt from the crimson, round bodies. The green leaves are beautiful, the red veins forming intricate spider web patterns. I bunch them together in groups of four with rubber bands and place them standing up alongside one another in a clean tub. The rain drums harder on the roof. I love that I am not thinking about anything else at this moment. In fact, for a while, I am lulled into a nice illusion that nothing else exists. I do not have to drive anywhere, run into traffic or crowds. I am immersed daily in the cornfields, blueberry bushes, zucchini and squash plants. And I love every single, solitary minute of it.

I finish scrubbing beets and then I help Andre check the corn for ear worms and snap off any pointed tips.

"So much of farming is rejection," he sighs, throwing away an ear worm-bitten piece of corn in disgust.

"What do you think art is all about?"

"No one knows more about rejection than I do," he says, with a laugh. "Seriously, people complain about this or that vegetable, the prices, the quality. In fact, one woman accused me of sitting around at market, collecting money. Yeah . . . I dream of the day I'll be making five dollars an hour."

"You've had a long day today."

"Yeah, I've had a long life," he says wryly.

"Do you love to do it? Would you do anything else in the world?" I ask.

He adamantly shakes his head no. "So I should shut up, right?" he asks, smiling wearily.

I grin. "Yeah. No, seriously, it's your passion to farm and you're pursuing it, regardless of whatever obstacles come your way. That's admirable." We finish checking corn and walk across the street.

Later before sunset, Scott teaches me how to seed lettuce. He scoops out a pile of mixed and sifted peat and compost, soaks it with water, and pats it down like a colossal mud pie. He demonstrates how to use the soil blocker, an efficient and impressive tool for starting seedlings. He pushes the soil blocker into the rich, fertile soil mix of peat and compost, then presses it into a tray and produces twenty cubes with holes of the proper depth for the lettuce seeds. He repeats this twice, and then I begin to disperse the lettuce seeds one by one into each of the cubes. I cover the tray with vermiculite, label it with the type of lettuce, set it aside, and start another tray until we have seeded sixteen varieties of lettuce. We carry them into the confines of the cool, damp basement to initiate germination. Hues of crimson and rose streak the sky while we clean up. I feel a sense of accomplishment; it has been a long, but productive day.

We end the evening walking through Newburyport, a Massachusetts seaside town. I had spent half my childhood, including a summer, at my grandparents in Rowley, about half an hour away. It is an evening filled with nostalgia, walking over the cobblestone streets and feasting on nachos at the Grog, a dark-paneled restaurant boasting walls of beautiful paintings and famous for its clam chowder. Scott shares some beautiful photographs he has taken of Andre's farm, and we talk of creativity, art, photography, and farming as an art. He wants to portray the seasonal cycles of farming and the evolution of Andre's farm. It is very much analogous to the evolution of a painting, the different stages of an underpainting.

We stroll around outside after dinner, pausing to listen to some live jazz emanating from a restaurant, the saxophone filling the August evening with its sweet melody. By ten, we are exhausted and drive home. I think I am asleep before my head hits the pillow later that night.

The steady drizzle of rain awakens me the following morning.

"I love to awaken to the sound of rain," I say to Andre over my oatmeal at breakfast.

"Yeah, once upon a time I did, too. But not as a farmer in New Hampshire," he says with a sour grin. It has rained, after all, almost consistently on a daily basis for the past month.

We start the morning harvesting zucchini, squash, peppers, and eggplants and hauling them in buckets across the street. My boots are not waterproof and soon my toes slosh around and wet pants cling to my legs, despite the rain jacket I am wearing.

"Farming is just as important as any other career in the world. It is equally as important as anyone else . . . doctors, lawyers, anyone," Scott says as we walk to the farm stand.

"I absolutely agree. Farming is a noble profession. You're providing everyone on this earth with food."

Where would we be without farmers? Farming seems to be a dying art and oftentimes, a scorned one. Yet, according to Thomas Jefferson, farmers were "the most valuable citizens." In Massachusetts, there are four times as many farmers over the age of sixty-five as under thirty-five.[3]

"Look at the twelve- to fifteen-hour days you put in, getting up at four a.m. to pick corn while the rest of the world lies in slumber, starting their day at nine."

"Hmph. I've been through half a day by then," he says, a bit of contempt crawling into his voice.

I laugh. "My mother yelled at me after I borrowed $25,000 in government loans to finish graduate school, then went to work on an organic farm for five dollars an hour. 'You are not a migrant farm worker' she yelled at me in exasperation!"

I reflect silently on this for a minute. So many people in the world make a living this way. I want to understand how hard they work, what the day feels like, how they feel at the end of each day. I love to sink my hands in the soil. I love the hard, physical, manual labor. I want to look at my vegetables and know how hard someone worked to pick them. I think everyone should at some point be required to farm, to harvest and grow his or her own food in order to sustain himself or herself. True sustainable living.

The morning is a flurry of activity, cleaning beets, bunching carrots, picking blueberries in the rain, and harvesting tomatoes in the greenhouse, while I swat away white flies swarming around me. We work feverishly until three and only because it is Scott's "day off," but he has bartered some time off so that Andre will repair the ball joints on his truck. Weary, we assemble some sandwiches in the kitchen, smearing homemade tahini and feta cheese on wheat bread, topped with tomatoes, red cabbage, and onions.

Scott converses with his mother on the phone for a while and hangs up, exasperated. He has decided to leave Rutgers and move to New Hampshire to pursue farming, far removed from the confines of the classroom. His parents are worried about him not having health insurance and giving up scholarship money. I wholeheartedly relate, having dropped out of graduate school three times and then pursued ecology, agriculture, and painting after graduation, none of which I learned in school. In fact, I had wanted to drop out of high school or at least go to a vocational school. I envied the students who went to learn car maintenance and repair, horticulture, and cooking. I had no intention of going to college, but my guidance counselor convinced me to try a year. Tony convinced me to finish.

"I don't want to be in a classroom!" Scott insists angrily. "If I go back, it is because I want to be there, not because I don't know what else to do. But I can learn what I need to know about farming right here, more than I can learn in the classroom. Maybe I'll finish at UNH, maybe I won't."

"So, follow your intuition. This isn't an irrevocable decision. See how you feel in a year. Maybe you'll finish in five or ten years. But so what? My brother left college at twenty years old and gave up a $60,000 scholarship to architecture school. He moved to Illinois to intern as a youth director at Stewart's church for probably what amounted to five dollars an hour. He had no money, no health insurance, but he was following a calling. And now at twenty-seven, he's finishing his bachelor's in theology and is a full-time associate pastor, preaching and leading his own worship service."

Andre walks into the kitchen and plops down in a chair.

"Just be prepared, Scott. You've led a pretty sheltered existence. Not having health insurance is the tip of the iceberg. Look at Amy."

"Thanks a lot!" I say and kick his chair.

"Sorry, but you're a perfect example, charging your rent and other bills on your credit card when things got really bad."

"That's what happens when you try to make a living from painting and writing—at the expense of jobs, money, and relationships."

Many people I have encountered believe that the financial and emotional suffering endured by artists, writers, and musicians for their passions is a *choice*. I will tell you that it is an inherent part of one's personality, perhaps even genetic makeup, and it is *not* a choice. I know many artists, writers, and musicians who experience great depression when they do not have time to create because of financial and family obligations. I am adding farmers to this list. I recently read an essay written by a farmer in *Sharing the Harvest* edited by Elizabeth Henderson. The farmer tried to explain his love of farming and concluded that he would farm down to his last nickel and would continue to farm until that was gone.[4]

"Would you trade it for a yuppie life of comfort and security?" Scott asks.

"Absolutely, unequivocally not," I say resoundingly. "I'd do it all over again."

"Do you want to know what I did last winter?" Andre chimes in. "I shoveled horse manure. I came home covered up to my ears in it."

"And he has a college degree," I interrupt.

"I finished college at twenty-seven, but I will tell you there are things I learned there that would have taken me years to learn on my own. Take Walter, for instance." Andre recently leased farmland across the street from Walter, a retired farmer. "Walter has a sixth-grade education and has educated himself. He reads incessantly. But he follows recipes, things he knows will work."

He does have a point. My graduate internships and education shaped who I am today and encouraged me to think and expand on theories in a thesis. To an extent, this degree is supporting my art and writing. Without graduate school, I may not have decided to work with adolescents or integrated environmental education and social work. In fact, this book would not exist were it not for the writing and research skills I gained in school.

Scott nods. "Thanks. It's really helpful to hear all this. I appreciate it."

"Whew, I don't know if I'm more tired from this morning or this afternoon's conversation."

He laughs and agrees. "Let's stop beating this to death and go to Fowle's." Fowle's is a cozy coffee shop in Newburyport, one I frequented when I was growing up. We spend the evening sipping chai tea and reading Robert Frost. "The Road Not Taken" has always inspired me to travel a less-trodden path in life, albeit one ridden with potholes and unforeseen obstacles around every bend.

I leave early the next morning, as I need to return to work and am anxious to paint and write. To my surprise, by the time I hit 495, tears well in my eyes. Is it possible for me to leave New England and not be brokenhearted? It is hard to make the transition back to work and reality after such an intense experience.

However, it is not long before I return again to New Hampshire. October ends with a long weekend at Andre's. A myriad of foliage blankets the land, the maples boast crimson red foliage, and the beeches bear leaves of golden yellow. It is an unusually warm fall morning, and my flannel shirt quickly absorbs the heat of the early morning sunshine. I soon peel off layers down to my thermal shirt. I am riding in the back of Scott's pickup, standing and trying futilely to maintain a foothold. He shifts into first and drives a few feet over the bumpy terrain, while I firmly grasp black plastic mulch from the ground and pull it into the truck bed. Black plastic mulch is effective for smothering weeds, maintaining warm soil temperatures, economical irrigation, increasing crop yields, and speeding up the ripening time of melons, eggplants, peppers, and summer squash.

Scott suddenly stops Blanchie Blue, his truck, named affectionately after Walter's wife. I lose my footing, lurch slightly forward, and grab on to the sides. He pokes his head out from the cab and looks at me, grinning.

"Very funny," I sneer at him but then cannot help laughing. He shifts back into first, then we proceed down each row, until the truck bed is filled with an entangled mesh of black plastic. We drive it over to a massive, wooden box. Scott jumps inside, and, in retaliation, I bury him with black plastic. He manages to escape, and then we zoom back into the fields to wind up trickle tape as the season is coming to a close. I encircle it tightly around my arm until I can see only my hand protruding from a large black ball. Trickle tape is used as an irrigation system and runs parallel in rows next to the crops. Water springs from punctured holes. We finish and drive back to the barn to place our supplies in storage.

"Let's go bag lettuce," Scott says. We walk down to the rows of lettuce. Beautiful red oak leaves beckon me to taste them and I bite into a crunchy leaf. I survey rows of green Boston leaf, endive, arugula, mustard, romaine, and radicchio. Scott pulls up the heads, and I snip off the excess stems, discarding them for compost. I spend the last remaining hour of the morning washing and bagging romaine lettuce, dunking the heads into a big tub of water, and rubbing dirt off the leaves. I cinch two heads together with rubber bands and slip them into plastic bags for market while Scott pulls carrots and digs potatoes.

Around 1:30, we break for lunch and walk across the street to the farmhouse. I smear some fresh goat cheese on homemade Annadama bread and scrounge around on the counters for a cucumber, red cabbage, and onions. I throw some diced slices between two slices of bread and wolf it down.

Temperatures soar into the high sixties after lunch. Scott disappears to spread rye, and Brandon and I work in the lower meadow, pulling up the remaining plastic and trickle tape. Brandon stands in the back of the truck, and I drive Blanchie over the furrowed fields. How exhilarating! I drive slowly down a row while Brandon pulls up plastic, and then shift into reverse, taking great care to avoid a nearby ditch, turn around, and drive down another row until the bed is piled high once again. We unload the plastic and then head over to the cornfields. Brandon whips out a machete the likes of which I've never seen. The blade glistens in the sun and, in one fell swoop, he deftly cuts the bottoms and the stalks plummet to the ground. I collect the stalks and throw them in the truck bed. We pile stalks until the rear cab window is no longer visible and then drive across the street. On our way out of the field, we see Scott driving a tractor and spreading rye. He looks radiantly happy, his hat perched on his head. He smiles and theatrically blows kisses. Brandon and I laugh, waving to him. What a glorious day to be driving a tractor!

At the farm stand across the street, Brandon demonstrates how to bundle the cornstalks, cinching ten together with twine at the top and the bottom, then stacking them upright in a row. Townspeople buy them as fall decorations for display on front porches. We finish in about an hour and then it is time to move on to bagging Yukon gold and red potatoes. Brandon explains the difference between ones and twos.

"Ones are the biggest and what you want to bag. Twos are smaller and we'll leave them for now."

He glances at a list.

"We need twenty five-pound bags and twenty ten-pound bags of golds. Same for reds."

I gaze at the sea of potatoes in front of us, piled in two old wagons. I am not talking about little wagons that children pull but of the old horse-and-buggy-style wagons! I start bagging golds in five-pound bags and place them on a nearby old-fashioned hanging scale. The needle teeters close to five. Brandon nods his approval, and I resume potato gathering. He glances over.

"Try to stay in one corner rather than going all over the place." Hmm. Sounds familiar.

"Let the potatoes come to you." He smiles and shrugs. "Least that's what Scott told me."

I laugh. "Sounds like Scott."

Through the open barn doors, I am startled to see that the sky is fading into darkness, the last hints of blue receding into blackness. We stack bags and bags of potatoes on the dirt floor of the barn until Scott comes in and tells us to quit. He backs up a truck, and we load potatoes; then he drives back to the farm stand. As I walk out of the barn, a gentle, cool breeze rustles the nearby hickory leaves. A silence has settled upon the farm, with the exception of a barn door creaking on its hinges as it bangs rhythmically against the side of the barn. The tractors are immobile, quiet statues of steel. I walk across the street to the farmhouse, listening to the gravel crunch beneath my feet.

Hilary whips up a beautiful ensemble of curried potatoes over basmati rice, and the aroma wafts through the kitchen for hours. We gather in the living room to eat and talk about the day. After dinner, Scott and I spend the remainder of the evening affixing his photographs of sunflowers, statice, leaves, sugar maples, and squashes to note cards to sell at the farm stand in the morning. We will be selling produce as well at an ecology festival in nearby Amesbury, Massachusetts.

The next morning we rise "leisurely" at eight, grab tea and coffee, and drive across the street to load Blanchie with pumpkins, bundled cornstalks, and butternut and acorn squashes. It is only a five-minute drive to the festival site, but I keep an eye through the cab window on the towering crates in the pickup bed. We arrive by 9:30, and, once again, temperatures are rising into the sixties. I jump out to help Scott unload, squinting in the brilliant sunshine. While we are unloading, I watch two llamas in a fenced area. Suddenly, one breaks loose and triumphantly gallivants toward the parking lot, dodging stands and gawking bystanders. I do not see anyone in hot pursuit of this runaway llama, but after the initial pandemonium, all calmly resume assembling their stands. Scott and I look at each other, laugh, shrug, and finish arranging the pumpkins, squash, and bundled cornstalks on makeshift shelves underneath the canopy. Scott posts his note cards on a board, and I prop up a few of my small paintings for sale. I recently completed one of a posterior view of Scott retreating from the fields, bucket filled with peppers, dressed in bib overalls and a rain hat perched on his slightly downturned head. It was a beautiful rainy morning, a fine mist enshrouded the fields, and the sky cast a whitish haze.

When we finish, someone announces the festival will begin with a Native American medicine wheel ceremony by the lake. Scott stays to tend to customers, and I walk to the ceremony, pausing along the way to talk to some exhibitors presenting environmental programs. I am very excited to see so many environmental education programs. I pick up some literature from Earthwatch, an organization that sends volunteers to work in the rain forest and other areas where volunteer efforts are needed. I finally reach the medicine wheel and join a long line. An elderly Indian woman dips a feather into a bowl and wisps of smoke curl upward into the air. She blesses each person as he or she enters the circle, gracefully waving the feather over the body in a crosslike pattern. I wait my turn and then am blessed. She motions for me to turn around and waves the feather over me. As it passes over my arms, I almost feel a gentle touch, and it is soothing. Feeling peaceful, I enter the circle formed by various stone structures. People who have already entered the circle sit on stones. Once everyone is inside, a young Indian woman plays a medicine flute, the melodic notes blowing in the wind. Another Indian woman softly says a prayer to mother earth, and an elderly Indian man steps forward to speak of a land preservation project. The ceremony is brief and closes with everyone holding hands. The woman who blessed us walks around the circle, hugging each person.

I walk back to the stand, where a friend of Scott's has agreed to stay and keep watch. We walk to the woods where there is an "art trail." Local artists exhibit paintings and sculptures along the trail. We stop to admire a bat hanging in a tree, constructed from scraps of discarded iron and steel, but the trees divert our attention, and we identify magnificent elms, leggy ashes, viburnum, cherries, maples, and greenbriar. We rest for a while, sitting on the edges of the trail, talking and watching the sun's rays filter down through the trees, casting a prism of brilliant light on the lake.

After a bit of time elapses, Scott needs to go back to the stand, and I wander through the woods a while longer, sit by the lake, and suddenly I hear the beat of conga drums. I jump up and follow the sound to the medicine wheel, and a Jamaican man with beautiful dreadlocks is drumming, his hands moving swiftly and methodically between two drums. Assorted drums are scattered on the ground, and many people are seated on stones, playing along, while others drift into the circle. Someone beckons for me to sit down and offers me a drum, which I eagerly accept (I had joined a drum circle while living in southeastern Pennsylvania). I stay for the next hour, happily drumming. Our dynamic and enthusiastic leader assigns various beats to random groups. At first, the tempo is a steady beat, but gradually it increases, culminating in an energetic frenzy of drumming. Just as I think I cannot drum any faster, it ceases. How powerful.

Guiltily, I decide to head back to the stand. As usual, I have lost track of time. Judging by the sun setting, it is close to five. Scott is loading Blanchie when I return. Some of the pumpkins were sold, but unfortunately quite a few remain. We attribute it to the distractions of the festival and drive home. On the way back, we stop at a farmer's market inside a handsomely constructed timber barn. Scott is mesmerized with the assortment of Liberty, Empire, Russet, Cortland, and Baldwin apples. He crunches into a "winter banana" apple and passes it to me. I bite into its firmness, the sweet juice oozing into my mouth. It does indeed hint of a banana. I had recently read of a fruit farmer in California who created a hybrid through open pollination called the "pluot," a cross between a plum and an apricot. We buy some apples and head home.

Andre and Hilary are peeling garlic in the dining room when we walk in. Crates of garlic bulbs are stacked in every available space, and garlic peels litter everything, including Andre and Hilary, who are hysterical and throwing the peels at each other. Mad farmers! Scott makes a couple of quick omelets for our dinner and helps me edit. Andre and Hilary soon join us, and they are in hysterics from reading this very chapter, especially my recollection of the septic system. Andre thinks I have portrayed him as a curmudgeonly farmer (I have) and myself as a sagelike person come to save him (perhaps), but I relent and agree to some editing (maybe). It is a good close to the weekend, and I enjoy sharing my writing with them. Sorrowful as always, I leave the next morning, disappointed I cannot stay and plant garlic.

Later that winter, we visit Bob and Jennifer for a long weekend to start tapping trees. However, the weather is not conducive to tapping; not one day climbs above ten degrees. One afternoon, Scott, Jennifer, and I traipse through more than two feet of snow up a mountain, our snowshoes gently crushing the fine powder. Despite the afternoon temperature of ten degrees, my long underwear, cotton duck workpants, and thinsulate-lined coat trap essential warmth. Clear blue plastic PVC tubing encircles the trunks, carrying sap down the mountain, propelled by gravity, to the tank in the sap house for boiling. Occasionally, a collapsed branch falls across a section of tubing, burying it beneath the snow. Layers of ice form an impenetrable crust, and Scott doggedly picks around it for a while. Once the ice breaks,

Jennifer and I salvage the tubing from the snow. Scott stretches the tubing and secures it tightly around the trunk. We trudge up and down the mountain, searching for broken or fallen tubing. Suddenly, we spot blue shreds of tubing randomly scattered across the pristine white snow.

"Squirrels!" Jennifer exclaims in disgust. She angrily shakes her head. "The snow's so high that they are sucking the sap right out of the tubes. It's too cold today, but we'll have to replace all of it."

She spots another broken section of tubing that is repairable and retrieves a new section of tubing from her backpack. She pulls it until the tubing is taut, and then holds the ragged end piece with her teeth, moistening it to attach it to the new section. Scott and I watch in fascination as she successfully attaches it. After this, she heads back in the direction of the house while Scott and I snowshoe for the remainder of the afternoon, observing the branches of sugar maples, green ash, Norway spruces, and white pines droop, heavily laden with snow. We snap pictures until my fingers are numb and then return to the house to help with dinner. After dinner, Bob plays the piano, and then we talk for the remainder of the evening. Jennifer and Bob's kids are away for the weekend, and we are offered a room in the loft upstairs. Snuggled in sleeping bags, we fall asleep under the "stars," fluorescent stickers glued all over the ceiling.

When I next open my eyes, frost has gathered on the outside of the loft windows. I listen to the bleating lambs and the roosters crow from the outside barn. Scott stretches and then walks downstairs for coffee, while I covet the warmth of the sleeping bag for a couple minutes until I drag myself downstairs for tea. The thermometer outside reads three degrees at eight o'clock in the morning. After a leisurely breakfast of eggs, toast, and tea or coffee, we snowshoe up Gore Road to glimpse the snow-covered peaks of Mount Kearsarge in the distance. Along the way, we examine some twigs and Scott shares his interest in Darwin's discovery of auxin, a plant hormone that is responsible for cell elongation on the darkened side of the meristem, causing a branch to turn upward toward the light. He has aroused my desire to study plant physiology, and, once I return to work, I enroll in an introductory crops course that covers plant physiology in great detail. (It is offered as an independent study course through the University of Guelph in Ontario, Canada.)

* * *

As I have become more involved with organic farming throughout the seasons, it has led to an inevitable change in my diet and lifestyle. The Greek physician Hippocrates, often referred to as the Father of Medicine by historians, believed in natural cures such as diet. Because of time constraints, Americans resort to diets of overprocessed foods high in sugar, salt, and fat. These lifestyles will inevitably lead to destruction of our bodies. My vegetarian diet consists mostly of organic food and my energy level has exponentially increased. I no longer have an annual case of bronchitis and strep throat. I don't know if there may be any correlations established specifically between organic food and ADHD; however, pesticides have been linked with hyperactivity and decreased academic performance. In the Mississippi Delta region, cotton is the biggest crop, requiring intensive doses of pesticides. A 1992 University of Mississippi study found consistently higher rates of cancer, infant mortality, low birth weights, and lower aptitude scores in students of the Mississippi Delta.[5]

Pesticides destroy cholinesterase, an enzyme critical to the central nervous system. Enzymes are substances that occur naturally in all living things: animals, plants, and human beings. There are more than 2,700 different enzymes in the human body. Through a complex series of chemical reactions, enzymes are catalysts in the metabolic process. In particular, neurotransmitters, such as dopamine, norepinephrine, and serotonin, are manufactured by the action of brain enzymes. A deficiency in enzymes may be correlated with low levels of neurotransmitters. The heat of cooking can kill enzymes. A fresh vegetable salad and/or steamed vegetables can alleviate this problem. Enzyme-rich foods include raw sauerkraut, fresh herbs, onions, garlic, and soy sauce.[6] Fresh fruits and vegetables are the best sources of enzymes. Papaya and pineapple, asparagus, figs, ginger, barley, wheat, rice bran, green beans, tomatoes, and oranges are other enzyme-rich foods. Eating only organic, pesticide-free food is one way to maintain and restore enzymes.[7]

All cholinesterase-inhibiting pesticides can cause adverse symptoms, such as *hyperactivity,* restlessness, neuromuscular paralysis, visual problems, breathing difficulties, and abdominal pain. Pesticides account for 2.1 percent of all U.S. cancer deaths each year, legally killing approximately 10,000 Americans without their informed consent. Pesticides (including soil fumigants such as methylbromide, insecticides, herbicides, fungicides, rodenticides, and nematocides) cause dizziness, diarrhea, headaches, tremors, vomiting, and weakness. Pesticide use has climbed to alarming rates, increasing thirty-three times since 1945. Approximately $7 billion worth of pesticides are used annually in U.S. agriculture; farmers apply nearly 550 million kilograms of pesticides to their fields in the United States alone.[8] Furthermore, forty-six different pesticides and nitrates from nitrogen fertilizers (used in conventional farms, not organic farms) have been found in the groundwater of twenty-five states, with the largest residues in big agricultural states, such as California and Iowa.[9] Fifty-five percent of this country's antibiotics are given to livestock, and bacteria build resistance to these antibiotics. Hence, certain antibiotics are no longer effective for human diseases. Chemicals and carcinogenic hormones (diethyl stilbestrol-DES) are also added to livestock feed.[10]

Meat could be produced in environmentally sustainable ways; currently it is not. Land degradation from grazing now constitutes one of the planet's most serious environmental problems; 90 percent of harmful organic wastewater pollution is attributable to U.S. livestock. Livestock produces 250,000 pounds of excrement per second. Such pollution destroys fish and shellfish in rivers adjacent to livestock areas through runoff. A recent study discovered 35,000 miles of polluted rivers in twenty-two states. In addition, a recent study concluded that cattle fed a grain-based diet harbored *Escherichia coli* 0157:H7, whereas cattle fed a forage-based diet, typical of pastured organic cows, did not. Most types of *E. coli* are not harmful and are normal bacteria in the gastrointestinal tract of animals and humans. However, 0157:H7 is a disease-causing strain that produces toxins which cause bloody diarrhea or even kidney failure in humans. In addition, red meat acts as a stimulant and increases cholesterol.[11]

Organic food is more expensive, but it accurately reflects the costs of small-scale farming. However, small-scale farms are losing to agribusiness. Large agribusiness companies are focused solely on productivity and are intent on forcing higher yields from the land in an ever-increasing attempt to dominate nature and to subdue the earth, regardless of the toll it takes on our health, as is evident in the increasing rates of pesticide-linked cancers. Small-scale farmers are also losing to developers. In New Jersey, 51 percent of farmland has been lost to development, with significant changes in agricultural output.

By 1993, less than 2 percent of the population was left on only 2.2 million farms, so few that the U.S. Census Bureau announced it would stop counting them. The number of farms fell again to 1.92 million in the agricultural census of 1997. Between 1987 and 1992, Vermont lost seventy-three acres of farmland a day. New York State lost farms at the rate of twenty a week and farmland at the rate of 100,000 acres a year for twenty years. According to the National Agricultural Lands Study completed in 1981, the United States was losing *one million* acres of prime cropland every year, or four square miles a day.[12]

Large-scale, conventional farms are subsidized by the government and are dependent on the economies of scale and cheap synthetic fertilizers. When a farmer uses commercial nitrogen fertilizers, the amount of thermodynamic work expended to apply it is seven times greater than the minimum amount of work needed to accomplish the same result by planting vetch. Vetch is a legume and cover crop that is planted in the late fall to protect the soil from erosion and depletion of essential nutrients. Furthermore, conventional farms do not have to account for some of the costs of their practices and can therefore sell produce at reduced prices. Conventional farms also use 18,400 BTU of energy, compared to 6,800 BTU of energy used by organic farms to produce a dollar of output.[13]

Eating food that is not in season also contributes to the demise of local farms. Stores in the Northeast used to carry Florida tomatoes in the winter; with the North American Free Trade Agreement (NAFTA), the tomatoes come all the way from Mexico. After a few more years under the General Agreement on Tariffs and Trade (GATT), apples from China may crowd out Washington State apples. Buying in-season, local produce saves the costs of transportation, processing, packaging, advertising, and nonrenewable fossil fuels required to ship produce out of season.

The loss of farms and rural communities is costing all of society its health, education, employment, and, ultimately, the earth. In the mid-1990s, 77.5 percent of people lived in metropolitan areas and 50.2 percent lived in large metropolitan areas. The number of farms in the United States dropped from 6.5 million in the late 1930s to 2 million in 1990, less than 2 percent of the total population. Each farm failure means a loss of three to five rural jobs.[14]

Many small-scale organic farms utilize hand tools, more expensive biological fertilizers, integrated pest management, and compost. No pesticides or herbicides are used. Composted organic soil adds the essential elements of nitrogen, phosphorous, and potassium. Compost, or humus as the end product is called, is the decomposition of moist and dry materials, consisting of animal wastes, vegetable and fruit peelings, twigs, and leaves, essentially anything that is readily found in nature. The rate of decomposition is based on the ratio of carbon to nitrogen (25:1). Nitrogen is derived from plants and vegetable peelings (green) and carbon from sawdust, wood chips, and twigs (brown).

Shelves in the typical supermarket aisle are crammed with fat-laden, packaged junk foods and it is not surprising that essential fatty acid (EFA) deficiencies have been documented in some cases of ADD/ADHD. EFAs are necessary for normal growth and development and are the major building blocks of cellular membranes surrounding every cell in the body, known as lipid bilayers. Cell membranes serve as an effective barrier to unwanted substances.[15] Fatty acids are the molecular components of fats and oils. The body cannot manufacture EFAs; they can be obtained only through the diet. Fatty acids are divided into three categories: saturated, monounsaturated, and polyunsaturated fats. Saturated fats are found in dairy, meat, and tropical oils and increase the risk of coronary artery disease, diabetes, and obesity. Monounsaturated fats, which are found in olive oil and canola oil, help protect the cardiovascular system, reduce the risk of certain metabolic disorders, such as "insulin resistance" and diabetes, and decrease the risk of cancer.

Trans fatty acids, which are produced during the hydrogenation of vegetable oil, are found in margarine, vegetable shortening, commercial pastries, deep-fat-fried food, and most prepared snacks, mixes, and convenient foods and may also increase the risk of breast cancer. Hydrogenation is the process by which vegetable oil is heated, exposed to a metal catalyst such as nickel or copper, and transformed into a more plastic, less perishable fat. This fat is then added to convenience foods, which permits them to sit on a shelf for months. By 1979, Americans consumed 10 billion pounds of fat and oil per year, of which 60 percent was partially hydrogenated oil.[16]

Hydrogenation decreases the EFA content of oils by rearranging the molecular bonds on fatty acids, transforming them into *trans* fatty acids. Untreated soybean oil is approximately 8.5 percent alpha-linolenic acid (LNA); the LNA content decreases to 3 percent when it is partially hydrogenated. *Trans* fatty acids raise low-density lipoprotein (LDL) cholesterol (bad) and decrease high-density lipoprotein (HDL) cholesterol (good). Americans consume from 5 to 10 percent of their calories as *trans* fatty acids; amounts greater than 5 percent can have negative health consequences.[17] Anything labeled "partially hydrogenated" contains *trans* fatty acids, a common ingredient in most packaged snack foods.

Polyunsaturated fats are divided into omega-3 fatty acids and omega-6 fatty acids. The primary fatty acid in the omega-3 family is alpha-linolenic acid, or LNA. The body converts LNA into eicosapentaenoic acid (EPA), which in turn is converted into docosahexaenoic acid (DHA). EPA and DHA are longer-chain omega-3 fatty acids found primarily in fish oil. LNA is a shorter, eighteen-chain omega-3 precursor found in green, leafy vegetables, flaxseed, canola oil, and walnuts. The primary fatty acid in the omega-6 family is linoleic acid, or LA. LA is converted into gamma-linolenic acid (GLA), found in borage and primrose oil, which is then converted into arachidonic acid (AA), also found in meat:

Omega-3 fatty acids: LNA → EPA → DHA
Omega-6 fatty acids: LA → GLA → AA

Omega-6 fatty acids are found in common vegetable oils, such as corn, safflower, cottonseed, soybean, and sunflower oils. The longer-chain fatty acids, such as DHA and AA, make up one-third of all lipids (fats) in the brain.[18] Debate remains concerning whether the nutritional needs of babies can be met by LNA alone or whether longer-chain fatty acids are also required.

Children with the highest levels of omega-3 fatty acids have the fewest learning problems. Researchers discovered that boys with ADHD have significantly lower levels of both EPA and DHA than those without the disorder. One study revealed that approximately 40 percent of children with ADHD have an omega-3 deficiency. Boys with the most abnormal behavior have the lowest levels of DHA and are more likely to be hyperactive, impulsive, anxious, prone to temper tantrums, and bothered by sleep disorders, including difficulty going to sleep and getting up in the morning.[19] Another study showed that mice fed safflower oil (omega-6) are more hyperactive than those fed perilla oil (omega-3).[20] Furthermore, John Burgess, an assistant professor of foods and nutrition at Purdue University, speculates that children with low blood levels of omega-3s may not be able to metabolize the required amount of omega-3s from their diets. The prevalence of cases of ADHD in the past fifty years in the West may be related to an increase in omega-6 fatty acids and a deficiency of omega-3 fatty acids in our diets. [21]

DHA, found in breast milk, is necessary for optimal development of the eyes and the brain, in particular, the structural development of retinal, neural, and synaptic membranes.[22] Breast-fed babies have more DHA in their brains and retinas than bottle-fed babies. Breast-fed babies have better visual acuity than bottle-fed babies and score higher on standardized tests of reading, visual interpretation, sentence completion, nonverbal skills, and math. However, the use of Bayley's Scales of Development to assess these skills is controversial, as the measures provide a quantitative description of the ages at which an infant attains typical motor, behavioral, verbal, and mental milestones. Studies have shown that Bayley's scores obtained in the first two years do not predict childhood IQ to any "useful extent."[23]

A deficiency of omega-3 fatty acids is also related to abnormal adult behavior, including impulsiveness and aggression, often symptoms of ADHD. Male monkeys fed a diet with a high ratio of omega-6 to omega-3 fatty acids (33:1) engaged in more slapping, pushing, and biting. Evidence suggests that omega-3 fatty acids can help reduce the low-level hostility that comes from the stresses of daily life. Donald O. Rudin, one of the first American physicians to treat patients with omega-3 fatty acids, gave two to six tablespoons of flaxseed oil daily to forty-four people with mental disorders. Within two hours of taking the supplement, patients reported drastic improvements in mood.[24]

Flaxseed oil is the richest source of LNA; one tablespoon contains approximately seven grams. Two grams of LNA daily is adequate. It can be added to salad dressings, soups, and sauces before serving. It should not be heated above 210 degrees, as it is highly unsaturated and more prone to oxidation by heat, light, and air. Flaxseed oil should be stored in the refrigerator and used within a couple of months; oil capsules can be taken as well. Capsules and oil may be found in the refrigerated section of many health food stores. Flaxseeds contain three grams of LNA per tablespoon; one tablespoon also contains three grams of fiber. Flaxseeds can be ground into a fine meal and added to breads, muffins, pancakes, waffles, cereals, and cakes. They can be ground in a coffee or food grinder (not a food processor) or purchased preground at a health food store.

Cod liver oil is not recommended as a primary source of omega-3 fatty acids. Cod liver oil comes from a cod's *liver,* an organ that accumulates high amounts of vitamins A and D. Vitamins A and D are fat soluble, which means that any excess amounts will be stored in the tissues. To get enough EPA and DHA from cod liver oil, one would have to exceed the recommended dosage. It is advised to take one gram of EPA plus DHA. Plain fish oil supplements are recommended as an alternative. Most studies were based on the use of supplements, not on the actual consumption of fish.

The body functions at an optimal level when the diet contains a balanced ratio of EFAs, yet the typical Western diet contains fourteen to twenty times more omega-6 fatty acids than omega-3 fatty acids. Since the 1960s, our consumption of omega-6 oils has more than doubled, making Americans the world's second largest consumer of omega-6 fatty acids, topped only by the Israelis. An ideal ratio of omega-6 to omega-3 fatty acids is less than 4:1, which was the ratio found in our evolutionary diet.[25] In his book, *The Omega-3 Connection,* Andrew Stoll, assistant professor of psychiatry at Harvard Medical School, recommends a ratio of 1:1 based on a recent national meeting of leading nutritionists, paleoanthropologists, cardiologists, psychiatrists, and lipid chemists. Fish, meat, fruits, and vegetables comprised the Paleolithic diet; cereals, breads, and dairy products were not emphasized.

A balance of EFAs in the diet also seems to influence the severity of depression. The traditional Japanese diet contains about fifteen times more omega-3 fatty acids than the American diet. Studies indicate that the Japanese have one-tenth the rate of depression of Americans. In the elderly population, contrasting levels of depression are evident as well; 44 percent of elderly Americans exhibit symptoms of depression compared to 2 percent of the Japanese elderly, with the lowest rates found in members of fishing villages. A pilot study found that omega-3 fatty acids might improve symptoms in bipolar disorder. Animals deprived of omega-3 fatty acids had significantly less dopamine and fewer dopamine receptors.[26]

Omega-6 fatty acids have been linked with cardiovascular disease and cancers. Oils high in omega-6 fatty acids send a message to the genes to produce more of a cancer-promoting protein called "ras p21." Omega-3 fatty acids render this protein inactive, possibly reducing the risk of cancer. Omega-3 fatty acids also instruct your genes to produce less of an enzyme that is essential for the production of fat and lower levels of a fatty substance called "triglycerides" in your blood, reducing the risk of cardiovascular disease. A study of 12,000 men on the Greek island of Crete found half the cancer rate and one-twentieth of the mortality from coronary artery disease compared to Americans. Ideal ratios of EFAs are found in the traditional Crete diet, which consists of large quantities of greens and wild plants.[27]

Certain wild plants, such as purslane, often considered a noxious weed, contain far more omega-3 fatty acids than cultivated plants. Purslane is loaded with omega-3 fatty acids; 100 grams contains 400 milligrams of LNA, fifteen times more than commercial lettuce. Purslane is rich in antioxidants; one serving fulfills the daily requirement of vitamin E and provides significant amounts of vitamin C, beta-carotene, and glutathione. It is the eighth most common wild plant in the world and one of the first plants cultivated by early humans. Originally, purslane seeds were discovered in a cave in Greece that was last inhabited 16,000 years ago. LNA is found in most dark green leafy vegetables, mosses, ferns, and legumes, as well as in many herbs and spices, such as mustard, fennel, cumin, and fenugreek.

Eggs of chickens that graze on wild plants are also rich in omega-3 fatty acids, compared to animals kept in confinement and fed an artificial, grain-based diet. It is apparent that some are aware of the need to return to this type of diet, evident in stores touting "free-range" meat. Free-range animals are allowed to eat a natural diet of wild plants. Greens, insects, and worms are the natural diet of chickens, not commercial cornmeal mash.

Sugar and caffeine are two of the most harmful substances consumed in excess by most Americans. Caffeine stimulates the nervous system, heart, and respiratory systems, thereby aggravating restlessness, and increases mood swings and irritability. One study reported that even moderate amounts of caffeine consumption can cause withdrawal symptoms: headache, decreased mental alertness, irritability, and fatigue. Refined sugar overstimulates production of insulin. Blood sugar thus increases and plummets, or "crashes," quickly, resulting in fatigue.[28]

Certain vitamin deficiencies have been documented in children with ADD/ADHD. In the presence of normal IQ, a magnesium deficiency may result in excessive fidgeting, restlessness, psychomotor instability, and learning difficulties. Sources of magnesium can be found in green, leafy vegetables and nuts such as cashews and almonds. Vitamin B_6 has been found to be more effective than methylphenidate (Ritalin) for hyperactive children and to improve behavior.[29] Niacin has been found to improve school performance and social relationships and to calm hyperactive children.[30] Significantly lower zinc levels have been found in children diagnosed with ADHD.[31] A substance called nicotinamide adenine dinucleotide (NADH) can alleviate fatigue and stimulate cellular production of the neurotransmitters dopamine, noradrenaline, and serotonin.[32]

Recently, I attended an agriculture and education conference at the Rodale Institute in Emmaus, Pennsylvania. It was distressing to hear that the least taught environmental programs in schools included *agriculture and society* and *humans and the environment.* I was under the impression that humans and the environment constituted the world. Should it be any wonder that vitamin and EFA deficiencies are rampant? That we are the world's second largest consumer of omega-6 fatty acids and that our children score low on aptitude tests? That Americans suffer from depression, a range of mental disorders, cardiovascular disease, and high rates of cancer? We have created the problems, but part of the solution to many of these calamities will be found in our diets. With proper nutrition education, schools can be instrumental in finding solutions by planting gardens, teaching nutrition, and serving nutritious, balanced meals.

During this conference, I had the opportunity to hear a lecture presented by Dr. Antonia Demas titled Food Literacy. Dr. Demas discussed a study of 560 K-12 students in Trumansburg, New York. During this study, the intervention group was introduced to sixteen different foods, including various ethnic foods, through activities such as designing recipes, cooking, and keeping food journals. The control group did not receive any food education. Upon conclusion of the study, the control and the intervention group gathered to eat a prepared meal and weighed the food prior to consumption. The intervention group ate *twenty times* more food. Obviously, the education and experiential participation enhanced their likelihood of trying foreign foods. Furthermore, they reaped social benefits from this experience. Exposure to other cultural foods increased the acceptance of people from other cultures, thus helping to overcome prejudice. The outcome of the experiment did not stop at school. The students also brought the results of their experiences home, asking their parents to take them to the store to shop for ingredients to prepare meals at home.

Study results concluded the following:

- Seventy-one percent of students cooked their recipes at home.
- Seventy-four percent of students reported that friends and relatives with whom they cooked liked the food.
- Eighty percent of students wanted the recipes served in the school lunch program.
- Ninety-one percent of students requested that the nutrition project continue the following year.
- Sixty percent of students reported that their eating habits improved as a result of the project.[33]

Other schools are recognizing the correlation between diet and behavioral problems. Dr. Demas also presented a case study of the Appleton School in Wisconsin, a population comprised of students convicted of rape and murder crimes. One year, they allowed students to eat only organic food. For the first time in eighteen years, the principal did not record any suicides, incarceration, or drugs; there were no dropouts after that year for the first time. An experiment revealed student satisfaction; the principal held a "junk-food day" and, expectedly, behavioral problems increased and students reported feeling dissatisfied with their behavior. Ironically, the school lost $100,000 of its funding. Is the interpretation that we only fund schools for detrimental behavior? Why are we not funding schools for organic gardening supplies? Presently, schools are contracting with McDonald's, Taco Bell, and Coca-Cola. Coca-Cola is offering $1 million dollars to schools who exclusively offer their vending machines, regardless that these products are pumping caffeine, sugar, and corn syrup into the bloodstreams of students. Is it any wonder that fatty deposits in arteries are being discovered in four-year-olds or that adult-onset diabetes is now afflicting children?

The Westtown School, a Quaker school housing prekindergarten through grade twelve, is situated on 600 acres, the only land left preserved in Chester County, Pennsylvania. Global crisis awareness is taught at the elementary level. Programs teach recognition of native plants and gardening, composting, soil science, Native American medicine wheels, and healing herbs. The Food, Land, and People project teaches the interdependence of agriculture, environment, and human needs and works to promote informed consumer choices and sustainable agricultural practices. It expands on existing programs and promotes agriculture and environmental awareness, critical thinking, and problem-solving skills.

Unfortunately, in the education system, including colleges and universities, agricultural programs are separate entities, evident even in the infrastructure. In 1862, the Morrill Act allocated money from the sale of public land apportioned to each state for at least one college to teach agriculture-related subjects. The Hatch Act, passed in 1887, created the state agricultural experiment stations, intended to ensure agriculture a place in research. In 1914, the Smith-Lever Act created the cooperative extension service to impart agriculture-related information to the public. Together, these acts comprised the land grant college complex, initiated by Senator Justin Smith Morrill of Vermont, who intended to preserve agricultural practices and education. However, agricultural campuses today are often isolated, perhaps banished to the perimeter of the university, and if any interdisciplinary programs exist, one can be sure that agriculture is excluded.

I conclude this chapter with an appropriate quote from David Orr:

> If agriculture might have evolved differently in a liberal arts setting, I think the inclusion of agriculture would have helped liberal arts colleges avoid the debilitating separation of abstract intellect and practical intelligence. Instead, we have developed a version of the liberal arts in which it is assumed, without anyone ever quite saying as much, that learning is an indoor sport taking place exclusively in classrooms, libraries, laboratories and computer labs and that practical competence is to be avoided at all cost. . . . [T]his leads me to propose that agriculture should be included as part of a complete liberal arts education, first because it offers an important kind of experience no longer available to many young people from predominantly urban areas.

Student responsibility for farm operations would teach the values of discipline, physical stamina, frugality, self-reliance, practical competence, hard work, cooperation and ecological competence.[34]

Chapter 5

Up on the Mountain

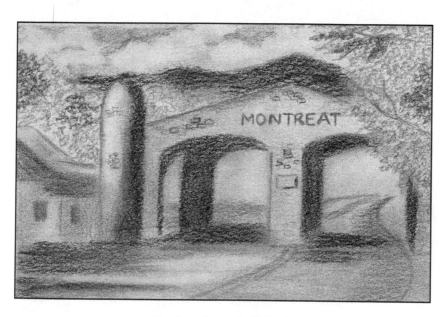

Seek and ye shall find.

Luke 11:9

How can I be of use in the world? Cannot I serve some purpose and be of any good? How can I learn more? You see, these things preoccupy me constantly.

Vincent van Gogh

My mother raised us Presbyterian; my father is a very reformed Jew. We attended a picturesque 200-year-old church in Princeton Junction, New Jersey, until I was seventeen. After that she gave up. Our Sunday morning conversations went like this:

"Are you coming to church?" My mother stuck her head in the door. This was a trick. It was not a question. It was an invitation to commence a battle of wills. I usually moaned and pulled the covers over my head.

"That's just great, Amy, just great. You know, God doesn't take off on Sunday for you."

"God doesn't also have to be at church by 9:30 after staying out late Saturday night," I retorted.

"Fine, Amy, fine."

"I don't need to go to church to believe in God!" Usually at this point, she slammed the door and left.

Until my twenty-fourth summer, I considered myself agnostic. Throw in Judaism, attend a private Catholic high school one year, and you get the product of one confused person who would prefer to abstain from any religious organizations.

My brother Chris, two years younger than I, became very involved with the youth group and eventually took over as an interim director between associate pastors. He volunteered his time, often putting in thirty hours a week while going to a community college. We did not have a formal youth group while I was growing up, and I now wish to have had the opportunity.

For six summers, Chris traveled to Montreat, a small town in the mountains of North Carolina, population 500, and host to the annual week-long youth group conference. Imagine 1,200 kids running amok in Birkenstocks and toe rings and this should yield a clear image of the week.

I had recently left my job as a group therapist with elementary-age inner-city children, as I found the routine intolerable. After four years, I was also laid off from my other job, working as a personal editorial assistant and helping to manage an estate for a writer. Unemployed and ambivalent about committing to any career, a thought popped into my mind. Go to North Carolina. I don't know where it came from, as I'd never gone before, but I called our associate pastor, Craig, who encouraged me to go.

* * *

Driving south a week later on Interstate 95 in a huge extension van with three youth group leaders and eight kids, I ask one of the youth group leaders what to expect.

"I can't tell you too much," she says. "You'll have to form your own opinion and it's better not to have any expectations anyway. It's so different for everyone."

A bit apprehensive, I settle into my seat for the ten-hour ride.

Soon after the sun fades from view behind the mountains, we drive through the Montreat stone gates and traverse winding roads on the Montreat-Anderson college campus. A van drives past us and a blond head emerges from the passenger window.

"That's Chris!" everyone shouts.

He recently moved to Illinois to intern as the youth director with our former associate pastor, Stewart. I know he will be surprised to see me.

We drive past Lake Susan in the middle of campus and around old stone buildings that dot the landscape. Pulling into Davis Hall, our assigned sleeping quarters for the week, we scramble from our seats and jump out of the van. We caravanned down with another church from Hopewell, New Jersey, and were meeting the groups from Illinois and Nassau Presbyterian from Princeton. My sister Rebecca, fifteen years old and also very involved in youth group, has come along for her second year. I run over to Chris, who looks at me, shakes his head, and blinks his eyes.

"What are you doing here?" he asks wide-eyed in disbelief.

"I kind of missed you," I say, hugging him.

Stewart also stares at me in shock and throws his arms around me. We spent many a late night conversing around our dinner table with Stewart and Bonnie, his wife, and they left a gaping hole in everyone's hearts when they moved to Illinois.

We mill around the parking lot for half an hour while Chris and Stewart get keys to the dorm. They return somber-faced and deliver the news: we are one night early and the college refuses to let us into the dorms. Moans and groans echo throughout the parking lot while a miniconference among the leaders ensues; we try Hickory Lodge down the mountain for the night.

Two hours later, fifty kids and ten leaders are safely ensconced in the one-story Hickory Lodge, an old log cabin with two bathrooms for sixty people and three people to a room with two beds. Someone places a massive pizza order, and we meet in the small lounge area to discuss the next day. Chris strums his guitar and leads us in songs while everyone clusters around him and demands his devoted attention.

Early the next morning, we dress and pack to move into the dorms later in the day. First, we hit a diner for breakfast, then church in town, and free time until the conference kicks off at 7 p.m. After church, we move into the dorms and distribute keys to the kids. Craig decides there will be one leader and two kids in each room. I am assigned a room at the end of the hall, and one of the girls approaches me.

"I assume you'll be taking one of the beds?"

"You assume correctly," I answer.

"I'm used to sleeping on the floor, anyway."

"Good," I say and cannot help the creeping edge of crankiness.

After I have a refreshing swim and make the near ninety-degree descent down the mountain to the dining hall for dinner, the Montreat conference officially begins. From the dining hall, everyone races over to Anderson Auditorium and stands at various doors, waiting to pounce.

I nudge my brother.

"Why is everyone doing this?"

"It's part of Montreat. You'll see," he says smugly. "We need to run in and grab five rows of seats for our group."

When the doors open, 1,200 kids push their way in and grab seats, almost trampling me in their haste. U2's "I Still Haven't Found What I'm Looking For" blares over a PA system, and everyone is singing and frenetically dancing in their seats. A guy sporting long dreadlocks waves a puppet on his hand. Someone tells me his name is "Tree"; he is a small-group leader. I am feeling somewhat hesitant and wonder if this is a born-again Christian cult. The dancing continues and the cheering increases as two people run on stage.

"Questionable Certainty!" they yell into a microphone. "That's our theme for the week. And as you divide up into your small groups tomorrow, you'll be hearing more about this. We hope you have brought a lot of questions, because this week will be the opportunity to ask." There was no shortage of questions I could ask.

The first speaker, Lona, is an attractive and petite Asian woman. She steps to the microphone and begins, "I never planned to become a minister. Both my parents were ministers, but I had decided not to become a minister. Sure, I'd always been active in church and I grew up in a youth group, but that was it for me. Then after I graduated college, I had no idea what to do with my life. I moved to San Diego, far away from my family, and I was feeling quite lonely. I prayed and asked God what to do. One day, for some reason, I wandered into a church in Mission Beach. I noticed a sign over my head, and it said, 'LO.' This was the nickname my parents called me and I decided that was as clear as it was going to get. I knew then that God wanted me to be a minister, and I got accepted into seminary next year."

I sit forward in my seat. She continues. "However, I was looking for a sign and I think people want a lightning bolt to strike them to help them decide what to do in life . . . and most of the time, people are so busy looking for a sign that they miss opportunities. . . . There's the old story about the man caught in a flood. . . . He climbs on top of his roof and cries, 'God! Please save me!' So God sends a life preserver and the man says, 'No, I'm waiting for God to save me!' Pretty soon, a couple rows by with a boat and the man calls out, 'Thanks, I'm waiting for God to save me!' A few minutes later, a helicopter whirls by and the man once again says, 'Thanks, God will save me!' Well, the man drowns and when he gets to heaven, he says to God, 'Why didn't you save me?' And God says, 'I sent you a life preserver, a rowboat, and a helicopter!' The moral of this story? Don't be so busy looking for signs that you overlook opportunities! Listen to God. What is he sending you that you may be missing?"

I sit back and glance around the auditorium, packed with youthful faces, meditative and intrigued. Am I so busy trying to analyze my own life that I'm closing my eyes to everything? I think about the plethora of opportunities that have arisen in my life. Lona finishes her sermon, but my thoughts wander as I think about how timely this message is. The service wraps up in prayer and song, and we leave for "icebreakers," which are games to help everyone get acquainted.

We head out to the tennis courts and someone yells into a microphone, "Walk around and find someone whose birthday is in December and then stay with that person!" A dull roar increases to ear-shattering decibels as everyone starts screaming and running around, forming groups. The games continue, and some of the leaders from our group break away and hang out on the far side of the tennis court. Chris finds a beach ball, and, for the next hour, we run around playing tag and slamming the ball into each other's faces. I fall on the ground clutching my stomach from laughing so hard, and Stewart, never one to miss an opportunity, pummels me with the ball. Finally, we walk back to the dorms, and I fall into bed, delirious from exhaustion.

The next thing I know, one of my roommates is shaking me.

"Amy! Come on, breakfast in ten minutes."

I pull the covers over my face. It cannot possibly be morning.

"The alarm hasn't gone off yet," I say, annoyed.

"It went off fifteen minutes ago," she sings.

I hear doors slamming in the hallway, music playing. I yawn, throw on a pair of shorts and a T-shirt, and stumble groggily down to breakfast. I find a seat next to Chris, who is already letting the food fall out of his mouth for a receptive audience of senior high school students. I polish off a bowl of cereal and then once again join the stampede to the auditorium for morning energizers. It's only eight o'clock. Energy and morning are not synonymous in my vocabulary, but it appears I may have to adapt this week. Once inside, everyone screams "Star Trekking!" and the entire auditorium begins to dance, pantomiming horns protruding from their heads and waving their arms in a flight pattern.

One of the leaders screams to me, "This is my favorite!" Feeling self-conscious, I join in, but everyone else looks silly and my self-consciousness rapidly fades. A couple more energizers and we sit down for our group assignments. Group leaders are assembled along the walls, and we are assigned numbers. I scan the wall and finally spot a short, blonde woman holding up the number 19. I bid farewell to my nearby seatmates and join my small group for the week.

"Hi y'all, my name's Laura. Follow me!"

We follow her outside to a remote spot, under a grove of pine trees. I nervously glance around my group, comprised mostly of high school seniors and several leaders from other churches. Stewart once told me to go where you feel most inadequate, a feeling that seemed appropriate at the moment.

"First, let's go around and just tell me where you're from."

I dread these introductions. In college, my fear of public speaking became so intense that the butterflies in my stomach fluttered long before it was my turn, my heart pounded, and I trembled when I spoke. I avoided and dropped any class possible where I had to give an oral presentation. By my senior year, I was desensitized enough by mandatory presentations, but I still vividly recall those days. I somehow manage to deliver my name, and Laura hands out our first assignment: draw our impressions of God. She gives us chalk to draw our impressions on the sidewalk and everyone starts drawing. Some people draw hearts, others draw male figures donned in robes, others draw peace signs. I hunch over, chalk poised over the sidewalk, a clean sidewalk. What is God? Who is God? I do not visualize God as a male figure or representing any sort of a person. God strikes me as an omnipotent presence or spirit blanketing the world. To symbolize this, I draw a square and completely shade it in to represent my interpretation of God.

Laura announces it is time for lunch, and I stand up and stretch, satisfied with my impression, albeit an ambiguous one. Does God appear as one dominant spirit or does He appear in a different form to each individual, based on his or her interpretation? Does God, as a spirit, only exist in our minds or is He someone we really meet and converse with after death? By using "He," I am not implying any concrete visual interpretation of God. Is an impression even worth our thoughts and time or should we solely focus on our faith? From my experiences, faith and Christianity are highly individualized journeys, involving pain, assuming much risk, and venturing into unknown territory. It is a calling that one opts to follow, or perhaps not; it often feels like stepping out onto a quivering tree limb to grasp another limb for the sake of jumping to another tree. You have no confidence that this limb will not snap and you will plummet to the ground; you simply take a leap of faith in hope of what lies ahead in the next tree.

My family and I attended a dynamic and powerful sermon that my brother preached a few days before the much-anticipated spring solstice. Intuitively, I felt I needed to hear him preach, and the words of wisdom he bestowed upon the congregation only reinforced this decision. He cautioned us to be prepared upon inviting Jesus into our lives, drawing an analogy of a house: If Jesus walks into your house after you invite him in, be prepared for him to clean out the drawers. Furthermore, you cannot cower on the back porch while he is inside. Essentially, do not ask for Jesus to come into your life and hide in the darkness, and then slightly step into the shadows. You need to boldly step into the glare of the light, for that is where you inevitably will be. Chris held up a newly printed T-shirt donned by his student ministries team. Scrawled in bold letters was *"jump first, fear later."* Not a simple depiction of Christianity, but a clear and concise one. He further elaborated on this in a vibrant song he wrote and recorded called "The Way." In *Mere Christianity,*[2] C. S. Lewis warned, "God is no fonder of intellectual slackers than of any other slackers. If you are thinking of becoming a Christian, I warn you that you are embarking on something which is going to take the whole of you, brains and all."[1]

Maslow defined "faith" as giving a meaningfulness to the universe, a unity, a single philosophical explanation.[2] C. S. Lewis defined faith simply as belief, in one sense, yet it is our imagination and emotions that often preclude our faith. True faith is maintained regardless of emotions or moods. Faith is nurtured, Lewis stated, through daily prayer, reading, church attendance, and practicing the virtues of Christianity over a lifetime. It is based on developing a trust in God and learning how to maintain that trust. Fully giving my worries to God has been one of my greatest challenges; it is no longer the struggle it once was but, nevertheless, remains a challenge, and I know I am not alone in this thinking. Prayer has helped to abolish this feeling, as has talking to others who share similar struggles. Lewis writes:

> Theology is like the map. Merely learning and thinking about the Christian doctrines, if you stop there, is less real and less exciting. . . . Doctrines are not God: they are only a kind of map. But that map is based on the experience of hundreds of people who really were in touch with God—experiences compared with which any thrills or pious feelings you and I are likely to get on our own are very elementary and very confused. And secondly, if you want to get any further, you must use the map.[3]

Many are seeking to fill a void, an existential cry to find meaning in their lives. Some accomplish this through addiction: alcohol, drugs, smoking, shopping, sex. I recall a sermon that Craig wrote about the onslaught of "self-help spirituality," not condemning it, but suggesting that it inherently becomes an addiction as well. We are all seeking to satisfy loneliness at one point or another. We fear loneliness; Buddhism encourages one to nurture or authenticate loneliness. It is, after all, an inevitable part of life. Avoiding it is analogous to hiding from death; it will find you, and it is good to be prepared for it.

We seek to fill these voids through psychotherapy. However, traditional psychotherapy may foster a sense of individualism, as critics contend that therapies focus on languages of self-interest and are destructive of the value of community in America.[4] People define their emptiness as an individual predicament.[5] Therefore, if psychotherapy continues to place an emphasis on individuality, will we not be perpetuating feelings of emptiness? If psychotherapy fails to fill this void, then people tend to pursue other avenues in the form of self-help books, addictions, and material possessions. Craig cited "mall spirituality" as an antidote to emptiness. Again, these "cures" focus on individualism and are temporary panaceas. What we are missing in our lives today is a sense of belonging, a sense of purpose, a sense of community and interaction with others. Our virtues of community are dominated by technology and the pursuit of wealth, contributing to our continued separation from nature, a loss that often creates emptiness. Churches, once an integral part of towns, arenas for social gatherings and dinners, formerly filled these voids.

In particular, churches need to reach out to the community and recruit disadvantaged and troubled youths. Youth groups are one solution for anyone struggling with ADD/ADHD, not only for youths but for adults who wish to become leaders as well. They provide an outlet for physical energy, a support system, and an introduction to mission trips and community service, as discussed in the next chapter. I did not have the benefit of a youth group in my adolescence, a resource that may have saved me a lot of turmoil and provided me with some direction when I desperately needed it.

Faith is the only thing that fills this void in my life. People are starving for faith in their lives, and it is faith that helps one to nurture loneliness. This is evident in those who seek therapists with spiritual values. A national Gallup survey revealed that two-thirds of respondents prefer to see a counselor who holds similar spiritual values and beliefs.[6] Another national poll revealed that nine out of ten Americans believe in God and consider religion important in their lives. Most Americans want spirituality, but not necessarily in the form of organized religion.[7]

Religion is typically associated with an external acceptance of a particular set of beliefs and ethics, and perhaps this may deter people from committing to prescribed values. Many may desire to explore different denominations, formulate their own set of beliefs, and then make a decision whether to commit to a particular organization. Spirituality may be, but is not necessarily, associated with organized religion.[8] Spiritual fulfillment may be found in music, poetry, literature, art, nature, intimate relationships, as well as religion. Spirituality may be waking up to watch the sunrise, strumming a guitar by a stream, or reading poetry in the woods. It is experiencing unification with nature and finding an inner tranquility. It is time for silent reflection on one's thoughts, and it allows our intuition, and thus wisdom, to develop.

"Spirituality" comes from the Latin root *spiritus,* which means "breath," referring to the breath of life. David Elkins writes:

> This involves opening our hearts and cultivating our capacity to experience awe, reverence and gratitude, the ability to see the sacred in the ordinary, feel the poignancy of life, to know the passion of existence and to give ourselves over to that which is greater than ourselves.[9]

For this to happen, we must relinquish our fears and tear down the walls of doubt and insecurity that surround us, that preclude us from achieving our potential and becoming "whole." This includes loving ourselves. Someone once told me that loving is the easy part; letting others love you is quite another story. One needs to first love oneself before having the ability to love another, as loving another involves both the giving and receiving of love. Therefore, one cannot receive love if one does not love oneself. Learning to love oneself may be accomplished through spirituality.

I ponder this for a while and then hike back to Davis for lunch. Dark, ominous clouds have gathered in the sky, hues of blue slowly blending into intensities of varying gray. Suddenly, a torrential rain erupts accompanied by a tumultuous vibration that quivers beneath my feet. Jagged lightning flashes, and people run for cover. I tempt the storm and avert my gaze to the sky, as chilling droplets trickle down my face. I kick off my shoes and carry them as I pounce into a puddle. The water splashes haphazardly over my legs, and I feel liberated. Another lightning bolt flashes and a roar of thunder accompanies it almost simultaneously. I stop playing in the puddles and run barefoot to the nearest building. A woman is standing on the porch.

"Come and get out of the storm," she says warmly.

"Thanks. I decided I'd better respect science and stop puddle jumping."

"I love to watch storms," she says, a contented smile spreading over her face.

"Yeah, so do I. I like to sit on my parents' porch swing and just watch the lightning."

"Where are you from?" she asks.

"Our church is in Princeton Junction, in New Jersey. What about you?"

"I'm from Cranbury!" she exclaims. Cranbury is a small town, close to Princeton Junction.

"It's funny to meet someone five hundred miles away who lives five minutes away."

"Yeah," she agrees. "It's a small world."

"Are you a leader?" I ask.

"Not at home, but I come here to help each year with the administrative stuff. Are you a leader?"

"Well, not really, but I'm here with my church, kind of tagging along with the students."

"What do you think so far?"

"How can I sum this up? I'm still trying to master Star Trekking, rebound from three hours of sleep, interpret God, and comprehend the power of prayer, all in one day."

She laughs. "It's only the beginning of your spiritual journey. That's a pretty good start. . . . Now you have the rest of your life."

I watch the rain trickle off the roof. "I'm at a loss of how I'll ever answer all my questions."

She wraps her arms around her knees. "Well, it won't happen today. Coming here is the best place to start. Montreat is a spiritual, magical place, this place up in a mountain . . . but what I learned is that you have to take it with you. . . . It's not just a place, but a way of life. I live on the 'spiritual high' for about a week when I get back to the real world, but it fades and I have to remember the feeling and kind of renew myself through other ways: in church, people . . ."

She pauses, and we sit in silence, listening to the drum of the rain on the roof that has decreased to a steady drizzle. I stand up and stretch.

"Thanks for the shelter . . . and the talk. I'll remember it when I leave. It was great to meet you. Maybe I'll bump into you someday in Jersey."

"You never know. Have a great week!"

"You too." I wave good-bye and walk to Davis to change into dry clothes.

As I walk down the hall to my room, Don, one of the students from another church, stumbles out of his room, crashes into the wall, and collapses on the floor.

I run down the hall and touch his shoulder. "Don!"

His eyes fly open, and he looks at me, startled.

"Where am I?"

"Were you asleep? Do you sleepwalk?"

"Yeah, sometimes. I came back to the dorm to take a nap."

I help him up and he walks back into his room and lies down on his bed, his matted brown hair clinging to his perspiring face. I sit on a chair, and I sense there is something more to this than sleepwalking.

"So . . . do you sleepwalk a lot?" I tentatively ask.

"Mmmm . . . I don't know. . . . It doesn't happen too often, every once in a while . . ." he says, looking up at the ceiling.

"Well, be careful . . ." I start to get up. "I'm going to change and walk down to the cafeteria. . . . Want anything?"

"Um, no . . . but wait a sec. . . . Will you talk to me for a minute?"

"Yeah, sure." I sit back down and wait.

"So . . . why are you here?"

I smile. "You mean earth or Montreat?"

"Montreat."

"That's a good question. . . . I have too many questions that I can't answer alone. I don't know, I think I needed something else in my life. . . . Why are you here?"

He shrugs. "I didn't have anything else to do."

"Aren't you in school?"

"No, I quit."

"Oh." I am quiet for a minute. "So, what do your parents think about this?"

"My dad's so drunk most of the time he can't lift his face out of his own puke."

He is quiet and looks at me, seeking something, perhaps some words of encouragement. "Well . . ." I begin. "What about your mom?"

"Gone. . . . She ditched us after I was born."

"I'm sorry," I say softly.

"Eh, it's no big deal. I've lived without her this long. . . . I've lived without a father, too, as far as I'm concerned."

"I'm sure you've heard this before, but can you go to Al-Anon meetings? There's always some at churches." Al-Anon is an organization for family members and friends of people suffering from alcohol-related problems. "I've heard really good things about the meetings, and you'll meet other people who are dealing with the same problem, and learn what you can do."

"I'm not going to some stupid group to talk about my feelings," he jeers.

"Well, can you talk to Kevin?"

He shrugs. "I've talked to him a little bit."

"Good, but you need to keep talking to him. Maybe give your dad some information about AA when he's sober one day, try to talk to him and let him know how you feel about his drinking."

"He doesn't care."

"Well, maybe he doesn't right now, but if you let him know that you care enough and want to help, it'll give him a starting point."

"Maybe." He crosses his arms in front of his chest and jiggles his foot.

"Do you work?"

"Yup, flipping burgers," he says, almost disgusted.

"So, it gives you some cash. In the meantime, maybe you want to look into getting your GED, do some stuff at church, go to youth group, and stay involved. Seriously, keep busy."

He nods. "I think I'll join the army."

"It might be a good experience—travel, education; you'll learn a lot. My dad was in the army and he worked as an illustrator. He's an artist, didn't belong in combat, so he got to do something he loved. You can't fight with a paintbrush, you know," I joke, trying to make him laugh.

It works. I stand up. "I'm going to go change and walk down to the cafeteria. Are you okay?"

He nods.

"Want the door shut?"

"Nah, thanks."

"All right, I'll see you later. Don't forget, we're having a paint fight at four."

"Okay."

I walk back to my room to change. I anticipate an interesting week ahead.

Later that night in the dorm lounge, Chris wanders over to a group of kids playing a game, leaving me with Stewart.

"Can I talk to you for a few minutes?" I ask.

"Sure," he says, sitting down and folding his arms across the back of his neck in typical Stewart fashion. Jokingly, he looks at his watch. "Go," he says, grinning.

"Today in small group, we were talking about God and my small-group leader asked us to draw our impression of God. Up until this point in my life, I've basically been agnostic; I don't even know if I believe in God. Suddenly, I'm questioning why I'm here, what my place in life is, who I am, how do I know what God wants me to do, does God have a plan for people, do things happen for a reason, do we have a destiny, and why does it feel as if God isn't answering our prayers sometimes?"

Stewart laughs and holds up his hands. "Whoa! This is going to take more than a few minutes. First, it's awesome that you have so many questions, and it's the greatest thing in the world for me to see people come to Montreat so full of energy and questions. So . . . where to start? . . . Well, does God have a plan for people? Hmmm . . ." He clasps his hands together and looks up at the ceiling. "Well, I don't believe in destiny."

"That reminds me of this debate I recently had with someone over this issue, someone who subscribed to the theory that our lives have already happened and we're just going through the motions." My adrenaline is charged and flowing, like someone has lit a match next to a butane tank. I sit back. "So, what do you think about that?"

"I don't agree. I think you may be born with certain talents and, therefore, you have certain choices to make in life based on those talents. I think you can ask God how you can best use your talents and ask for guidance."

"So what do you think about wrong choices, or really what society perceives to be wrong choices?"

"Well, that's a tough question, but again I think that people own the ability to make wrong choices, and that is called sin. God can't make you pursue a certain path, but He can help you. The Bible clearly defines sin and we, as humans, sin. But, you can also ask for forgiveness once you accept Jesus Christ into your life. What people need to do is invite God into their lives and pray about it."

C. S. Lewis addressed this in *Mere Christianity:*

> God created things that had free will. That means creatures which can either go wrong or right. Some people think they can imagine a creature which was free but had no possibility of go-

ing wrong. I cannot. If a thing is free to be good, it is also free to be bad. And free will is what has made evil possible. Why then, did God give them free will? Because free will, though it makes evil possible, is also the thing that makes possible any love or goodness or joy worth having.10

Stewart's answer does not quell my line of questions. "So, you do not believe in any destiny?"

"No, not in the sense that most people believe destiny to be. It comes down to what talents you have and those talents influence your direction in life. Like I said, you can pray for guidance, however, and ask God how to best use those talents. You know, God might have a general direction for you to go in. He might say, 'Well, Amy, I think you'd be best here'." He points to an invisible point in the air. "However, you may be down here, holding your hands up saying, 'God, I don't know what you want me to do.' Well, you make some choices, opportunities come along, and you wind up over here." He points to another spot in the air, below the first one. "Okay, so now you're a little closer. You feel like you're heading in the right direction, but you're still not where God thinks you can be. So, maybe God adjusts this point, and you wind up over here," he says, pointing to another spot parallel to the last one. "So, it's close to what God thinks is best for you, based on your abilities."

I sit forward. "So do you think some things happen for a reason?"

He nods. "I do. But, I don't believe everything happens for a reason . . ."

"So what about horrible, tragic things like someone getting shot?"

"That's sin. God did not create sin, man did. God didn't put a loaded gun in someone's hands and instruct him to kill another person. But sometimes amazing things happen out of tragedy—people become motivated to create changes in the world, restructure their lives, renew relationships."

I quietly mull this over for a while. "Does God answer every prayer, and are there things that you shouldn't pray about? Like things that would be misconstrued as greed?"

"You can pray to God about anything. You can pray to God you win the lottery!"

I raise my eyebrow and grin. "Oh yeah? Too bad I don't play."

"Well, if you did, it doesn't mean that you will win, but you can ask God for it. It doesn't make you a bad person."

"So, what if I ask God for something and I don't get it?"

"Well, God does answer every prayer in His time. And our time is not the same as God's time. Sometimes people are looking for an answer they want to hear and they miss God's answer because it isn't what they want to hear. That's the key. God may have something different in store for you, and it may not always be what you think you want. Do you see what I mean? See the difference?"

I slowly nod. "That makes a lot of sense. So I may want something, like a certain relationship to work out, but God may not think it's best. So, essentially, He is answering my prayer; it's just not the answer I'm looking for."

"Yup."

"So how do I know when God is answering my prayers?"

"Well," he motions around the room with his hands. "I think God answered one of your prayers. You're here, right?"

Chills creep over my body, and I sense this conversation has taken place for a reason.

He continues. "Your twenties are the time of greatest transition."

"Tell me about it. My life is suddenly unraveling, or, really, I'm trying to unravel it. I'm running in circles, spending so much time trying to figure everything out."

"You may not always trust God's hand, but trust His heart."

I want to soak in this moment of revelation, absorb it like a sponge, and bottle it to take home. And God is here, on this mountain. But He does not exist solely on this mountain or in Montreat. He always walked with me, but I never stopped and took the time to listen to His footsteps and acknowledge His existence, His power, His presence in my life.

Stewart clasps his hands in his lap. "Well, Amy, I sense that you're ready for this, and when people come to this point in their lives, I ask them if they're ready to accept Jesus Christ into their lives. I'll pray with you to do that. Are you ready to do that?"

I nod, without hesitation.

He bows his head and prays. "God, I thank you for bringing Amy here, for all her questions and curiosity, for our conversation. I ask that she opens her heart to you and invites Jesus Christ into her life. Amy, do you accept Jesus Christ into your life?"

"I will and I do accept Jesus Christ into my life."

"God, I ask this in your name. Amen."

"Amen." I am close to tears at this point, and we stand up. It's almost midnight, and the lounge is empty. Stewart hugs me.

"Thanks," I whisper. "Thank you for everything."

"You're welcome. I'm so glad you came."

"I am, too."

"Goodnight, Stew."

"Goodnight, Amy."

I head up the stairs and crawl into bed. My two roommates are sleeping, snoring heavily. I start to feel myself slip into unconsciousness and gratefully fall into the depths of slumber.

It is Wednesday night, and everyone at Montreat gathers around Lake Susan. A cool breeze blows across the lake, and I fold my arms to keep warm. I stand with my back-home group, holding an unlit candle. Suddenly, candlelight spreads around the lake, and I am mesmerized, watching this unfold. Wendy, a leader, taps me on the shoulder. I turn and tilt the wick to catch the flame from her candle.

The entire lake is now surrounded in candlelight, and the air is warm. I watch the candlelight cast shadows and illuminate the faces of those around me with whom I share this night, and all fears of isolation abandon me as we huddle together and sing for several more minutes. We begin to disperse slowly and walk back to the dorms. I cup my hands around my flame, shielding it from the breeze, composing a poem in my head: *Immersed in darkness, paralyzed with fear, I was hesitant to walk blindly into the night. Molten droplets cascade down the base of the candle, slowly trickling over my hands numb to pain. No longer hesitant, I walk on boldly into this vast, luminous night.* I sing softly under my breath in unison with those around me. Only when we are just outside the dorm do I allow the breeze to extinguish the flame. I walk upstairs to my room and carefully pack my candle in my suitcase.

Back in the dorms, chaos ensues as shaving cream fights break out, coating the walls white and creamy. Craig and Chris steal mud masks from the girls and paint their faces in blue, jumping in and scaring any unsuspecting people in their rooms. I flop onto Chris's bed and relate my conversation with Don to Chris and Stewart who are sitting on the floor.

"What do you guys know about Don?"

Stewart folds his arms and frowns. "Well, I know that Kevin brought him along to kind of help him out. He's had some pretty rough times."

"Yeah, so I've heard." I relate the conversation and sleepwalking incident. Stewart assures me that I did what I could and also agrees that the "sleepwalking" incident may be a ploy for attention. Kevin walks in midway through the conversation.

"I'll talk to him. I'm sorry you had to get involved."

"No, it's not a problem."

"Well, it is. I feel bad because I brought him here to help him out, and I didn't want other people to have to get involved. Thanks for letting us know about that. I think things are getting worse at home, and, yeah, I think it's a ploy for attention."

"Yeah, okay," I agree. "That's the impression that I got."

Chris looks at me. "So, are you glad you came?"

"If I had known all I'd have to do is travel 500 miles to learn all I've learned in the past few days, I'd have come a long time ago."

"Yeah, but you wouldn't have wanted to come then."

"I suppose you're right. So this is your life, huh?"

He grins. "This is my life. Never knew I was so great, did you?"

"How could I? You're my brother. I've lived with you too long."

The next day in small group, standing outside in a parking lot, we talk about trust.

"I want y'all to form a big circle," Laura shouts, flailing her arms about. "Now, turn around and look at the person behind you. Turn back around. On the count of three, without looking, the person behind you will yell 'Fall!' Fall backward. The person behind you will catch you in their arms. One, two, three!" People scream in unison, "Fall!" Everyone starts falling and then breaking into hysterics as some people collapse on their partner, bringing both to the ground, while others only "partially" fall backward.

"The purpose of this exercise is to get you to think about who you trust. First, you need to trust God." She retrieves a Bible from her knapsack and flips through the pages. "Romans ten, fourteen to fifteen. 'How can people call for help if they don't know whom to trust? And how can they know whom to trust if they haven't heard of the One who can be trusted? And how can they hear if nobody tells them? And how is anyone going to tell them, unless someone is sent to do it?'" She pauses.

"So, how many of you were afraid to fall back because you didn't trust your partner to catch you?" Many raise their hands.

"It's a scary feeling to completely trust someone to catch you, isn't it? But we need to first trust God with all of our hearts before we can trust others. Only then will you know who to trust."

"So," someone pipes up, "what if you trust someone who deceives you? Like here, what if I trusted my partner to catch me and he didn't?"

"Well, that's a good question. What do you guys think?"

A girl volunteers. "I believe that person who didn't catch you doesn't trust in God; therefore, that person doesn't trust other people either, right?"

Laura nods her head. "I think that's a very good answer. Anyone else?"

Another youth raises his hand. "I don't believe that you can trust everyone in the world. I think there are some people who are inherently evil, who don't love God. I myself just have a sense of who I can trust and who I can't."

"Is that something that happens over time and from experience?" Laura asks.

The guy nods. "From my own experiences, yeah. You kind of weed out people, I don't know, by intuition, I guess."

We continue to debate for a few minutes, then break for lunch. The afternoon is a free activity, and I hike in the mountains with Chris and some of the kids. After scrambling over a few rocks, we reach Lookout Point at the summit within an hour. The view, a labyrinth of green valleys and hills, steals my breath. The natural beauty is mesmerizing, so remote from the rest of the world. I want to live on this mountain, forever, far, far from the world. No one speaks, I think, out of fear of interrupting this revelation of God's creation. I walk over to sit down on a boulder jutting from the side of the mountain. An eagle flies by, soaring effortlessly over the valley. What it must be like to fly! The freedom, independence, exhilaration of flapping wings and lifting off the ground to soar over mountains and forests, exploring niches and crevices never explored before! I envy the eagle; my wings are broken. Yet I feel a sense of healing, awakening, and I want this power to fly, soar, and explore. A voice breaks into my thoughts, and I reluctantly get up and tear my eyes away from the mystic beauty. We begin the descent, single file, through the forest.

Abraham Maslow, one of the founding fathers of humanistic psychology, describes these transcendental "peak experiences" as revelations or mystical illuminations, and all, or almost all, of us are capable of experiencing them. During a peak experience, the whole world is perceived as an integrated and unified whole; one has a sense of belonging or place in the world. The experience may alter one's character and provide spiritual faith. From my experiences, it is simultaneously a dissociative state and a feeling of oneness with the world. Maslow referred to this as the cognition of being, or B-cognition. I believe that people with ADD/ADHD are more prone to peak experiences. Artists, writers, and musicians who possess high levels of creativity are easily distracted by a brilliant sunset, the sunlight glistening on a lake, an insect serenade under the moonlight . . . thus, the gift of paintings, music, poems, and books we all cherish. Maslow addresses the power of such experiences: "It is my strong suspicion that even one such experience might be able to prevent suicide and perhaps slow self-destruction—alcoholism, drug addiction, addiction to violence—may abort an existential meaningless."[11]

Maslow believed that nonpeakers fear losing control and rationality; therefore, they suppress and avoid these experiences. LSD and psilocybin can induce peak experiences, thereby granting an illusion of control over them instead of waiting for them to occur by good fortune.[12] However, this involves the art of developed patience. Patience can be developed through meditation, and meditation may possibly change our perceptions of life and increase our susceptibility to experiencing peak moments. According to Maslow, people who reject conventional religions, who develop private religions from their own private revelations, are more prone to peak experiences. Maslow believed that conventional religion tends to "dereligionize" other aspects of life. Practicing religion one day a week within a particular structure may absolve one of the necessity or desire to feel these experiences elsewhere. There are two sides to this. On one hand, I agree with this philosophy. I visit my brother's church on occasion to hear him preach, but I am not committed to any religious organization.

On the other hand, I have seen the benefits of belonging to a religious organization, having grown up in a church, as well as spending the first five years of my life in apartments for seminary students. My mother states that a burning ember dies once it is thrown away from the fire; there is truth to this statement. Mission trips and community service events created eternal bonds and lifetime memories; sharing my newfound faith with others strengthens it, and it is harder to maintain when I am "away from the fire." Singing "Silent Night" on Christmas Eve at midnight in the glow of candlelight is a magical, beautiful moment, shared with people I have known for twenty years. My father committed several years to volunteer monthly on the youth committee once my brother became active in the youth group. Participation in organized religion provides social support; social support in turn has been shown to enhance recovery and reduce depression in cancer patients. Cardiac patients had lower mortality rates six months after surgery as a result of participating in social or community groups.[13] Furthermore, a recent poll of 1,000 adults revealed that 79 percent believed that spiritual faith can help people recover from disease.[14] In a survey of 269 family physicians, 99 percent believed prayer, meditation, or other spiritual and religious practice can be helpful in medical treatment.[15]

I have personally seen the benefits of organized religion recently, when my twenty-eight-year-old brother Chris had a brain tumor surgically removed. His church collected enough money to pay for a hotel room for four nights close to the hospital, saving us the inconvenience and added stress of traveling two hours every day. Throughout his extended hospital stay in the intensive care unit (ICU) due to seizures following the surgery, a steady stream of visitors provided him with encouragement. Once he was discharged from the hospital, innumerable people volunteered as drivers after he suffered seizures from the surgery. People from his church came to the hospital for the long and arduous wait during his surgery. On the Sunday prior to his surgery the next afternoon, Chris preached his last sermon. He had written a song about the experience he had endured. During the final lyrics, he could not repress his tears; he walked down to where we sat and covered his face with his hands, sobbing. During communion, every single person in the congregation (probably 400 that day) walked up to him, many crying, and hugged him. After the service, many adolescents from his youth group gathered to shave their heads along with him in preparation for the surgery. About twelve people shaved their heads, including two women, one with blonde locks that fell to her shoulders. That night, while we had dinner together as a family, the church held a two-hour prayer service for him and our family. Irrefutably, this social support expedited his recovery. Four weeks later, I attended his church service with him. Everyone stood up and applauded when he led prayer, the only role he could play due to postoperative fatigue. The atmosphere was joyous and one of celebration, the antithesis of the gloom and fear we had felt four weeks prior.

What if one seeks a religious organization and comes away having not found fulfillment? Many seek solace in religious organizations and are disappointed not to find *immediately* anything that resonates with them. They stay reluctantly, unhappily, or leave unhappily. People are not finding any fulfillment because they do not have solace within. Perhaps they do not have a sense of community and thus lack a sense of belongingness, as explored in greater detail in the next chapter. Christianity, or any religion, is a journey where one constantly questions and seeks answers; it requires one to have learned the difficult lesson of delay of gratification. Delayed gratification is not taught in society today, clearly evident by the innumerable corporations peddling their wares and preying on consumers' desires and impulses.

Our last night in Montreat we gather in the lounge to sing and bid farewell. Chris strums his guitar and teaches us the lyrics of the song "The Mountain" by Steven Curtis Chapman:

> You bring me up here on the mountain
> For me to rest and learn and grow . . .

I cannot help the tears that spring to my eyes as I think of Lookout Point. "The Mountain" is a conglomeration of my experiences and feelings about Montreat. When Chris strums the last chords, I hear a few sniffles. Stewart stands up, holding bags of bread.

"I want each of you to take a slice of bread. Go up to at least five people, break off a piece and thank them for anything, any positive quality."

Everyone rushes to Stewart, grabbing bread and running up to people. Some of the kids are randomly tearing bread, yelling "Thank you!" to one another, while others are holding quieter conversations in corners of the room. I spot Don, a forlorn figure in the middle of the room. I walk over to him.

"So where's your bread?"

He sheepishly shrugs. "I don't know. Who am I going to talk to?"

"Go get some bread." He narrows his eyes at me but walks over to the abandoned, crumpled bags of leftover bread on the couch. I tear a piece off my bread and give it to him when he walks back.

"Thanks for having the courage to share with me what you did. A lot of people wouldn't talk to anyone, so I give you a lot of credit."

"Yeah, right." But he smiles.

"Yeah, right! I wouldn't say it if I didn't mean it."

"Thanks," he says quietly.

"Anytime. Just make sure you keep talking to people, okay?" He tears off a piece of bread and awkwardly holds it out to me.

"Thanks," he says again, only this time he enunciates it clearly, stronger, then turns to someone else, ripping off another chunk of bread.

I can't hold back my smile as I, too, tear off another piece of bread and turn to someone else. This continues for another few minutes and eventually some of the kids wander off to convene into groups.

The next morning is pure pandemonium, as we try to stuff forty-five kids in four vans along with assorted duffel bags, pillows, and knapsacks. Somehow, we achieve what seems an impossible feat and hit the road. As we pass through the stone walls that surround Montreat, I sadly glimpse back, savoring the moment. I gaze out at the fields, which quickly blur together as we gain speed, then finally reach the highway. Once we return home, Craig asks me to be a volunteer youth leader. Without hesitation, I agree, without any knowledge of the five-year journey that lies ahead.

* * *

The Council on Social Work Education and the *Diagnostic and Statistical Manual of Mental Disorders* of the American Psychiatric Association acknowledged the importance of spirituality for clients in their most recent curriculum policy statement. Many studies have also appeared in the professional literature advocating for the inclusion of spirituality in both social work practice and education. Conflicts arise because of the dichotomous relationship between counseling and spirituality due to the separation of church and state, the scientific method, the secular approach to medicine, and the agnosticism of Freud.[16] The challenge is how to transcend these obstacles. On the secular level, progression is evident, as nearly thirty U.S. medical schools now include courses on religion, spirituality, and health in their curricula.[17]

In a study of Israeli prisoners exposed to a daily routine of prayer and Jewish studies led by rabbis, only 8 percent returned to prison, compared to 67 percent of the general population of released prisoners who were reimprisoned.[18] The success of the resocialization and commitment to religion was, in part, attributed to the leadership exhibited by senior prisoners. Furthermore, the more time and energy one invests in a group, the greater one's sense of commitment to that group; one may adapt behavior coincident to the accepted norms of the group.[19] These findings may be generalized to adult youth leaders who hope to ignite a spark of interest in religion in resistant youths.

Carl Jung stated that spirituality was such an essential ingredient in psychological health that he could heal only those middle-age people who embraced a spiritual or religious perspective toward life. Erik Erikson believed that spirituality and religion play a potentially important role in child development. Belief in a benevolent and loving deity supports a child's sense of trust and builds a personal value system.

Many have lost a sense of spirituality and thus a connectedness to the earth. God created this earth, yet many have lost their connection to it, as they are consumed by technology and in the pursuit of wealth and material possessions. Similar to the severed ties between the food and health care industries, thus has been the relationship between Christianity and ecology. Revelation 11:18 states that God will "bring to ruin those ruining the earth." We have inevitably lost our sense of respect for the earth and ultimately ourselves. In his widely published essay "The Historical Roots of Our Ecologic Crisis," historian Lynn White stated that Christianity has insisted "it is God's will that man exploit nature for his proper ends."[20] Unfortunately, this has been translated as domination by man, which leads to exploitation and destruction of natural resources. Inevitably, this leads to destruction of our emotional and physical health, as well as our spirituality. White states that since the roots of our troubles are religious, the solution must also lie in religion. In a variety of published rejoinders, a sage presented an intriguing view: "Adam was created at the end of the sixth day so that if human beings should grow too arrogant, they may be reminded that even the gnats preceded them in the order of creation." [21]

If churches or other formal and nonformal religious organizations can restore these severed ties, whether through gardening, hiking, or any activity in nature, then we may begin to restore our severed ties to God and nurture our faith as well as our relationships with one another. Native Americans speak of a web of life and place emphasis on the interconnection and relatedness of events in our lives. Without a doubt, this should include the inherent relationship between religion and ecology. If nature intrinsically provides healing, churches should indisputably recognize a responsibility to instill environmental ethics that serve a dual purpose: reconnecting people to the earth for healing purposes and encouraging a sense of gratitude for the gifts of food and trees that grant oxygen to sustain our bodies.

Eastern religions focus on an intrinsic relationship with the earth. In the Hindu religion, trees and rivers are a powerful symbol of abundance and sustenance, as is evident in conservation efforts, poetry, and literature. Meditation and daily worship focus on the five great elements: earth, water, fire, air, and space. Yoga is practiced as one model of Hindu spirituality to enhance the body and senses. The doctrine of Dharma emphasizes the need to act for the good of the world. In South Asia, as environmental degradation increases, religious thinkers and activists contemplate the values of Hindu traditions.

Buddhist environmentalists contend that mindfulness produces compassion for all forms of life, especially for all sentient beings. This compassion is based on an understanding that all life-forms are interdependent. Today, Buddhist activists are addressing international issues such as nuclear waste disposal, human rights violations in Myanmar, and a peaceful resolution of the Chinese occupation of Tibet.

Christian theology is finally focusing on an ecological reformation that stems from a failure to acknowledge the interdependent relationship between humankind and nature. New insights will be gained through reinterpretation of the Bible in the context of contemporary society.[22] For instance, Psalms celebrates nature and the earth given to us by God with all of its beauty and resources that grant us sustenance to live. Christians speak of accountability for one's sins, but what about accountability for the earth God has given us? This in turn is accountability to God and to one another. When we pollute our rivers and spray our crops with toxic chemicals, we destroy ourselves and avoid any accountability. Why, if it is so clearly stated in Scripture that the earth sustains us, do we participate in such environmental degradation? Why does Christianity not integrate some of the values of Hinduism, Islam, and other religions? It is not defamation to one's religion to integrate the values of another if they are beneficial. Psalms 36:8-9 states, "We feast on the abundant food you provide; you let us drink from the river of your goodness. You are the source of all life, and because of your light we see the light." The Parable of the Sower in Luke 8:4-15 is an *agricultural* analogy referring to the seeds that are scattered as the word of God. The seeds that fall onto good soil represent those who hear the message and persist until they bear fruit.

In mainstream Christian churches today, environmental ministries are beginning to encourage an active discussion of planetary stewardship and creation spirituality. Churches and businesses "adopt" streams and beaches as components of their community participation programs. Since the 1960s, it has been assumed that environmental concerns belong to the Left without a thought of religious organizations playing a role.[23]

In 2001, I had the good fortune, through work, to attend the tenth annual Pennsylvania for Sustainable Agriculture (PASA) conference. One of the seminars I attended discussed religion, ecology, and sustainability. During this seminar, I learned of an event that had taken place in the spring of 1992. Religion and Science for the Environment organized a meeting in Washington led by religious leaders and science representatives to reflect a growing interest in environmental issues by the religious community. Over 3,330,000 congregations were represented, including the U.S. Catholic Conference, the Southern Baptist Convention, and the National Council of Churches. Senior Jewish, evangelical Christian, and Native American leaders were also present. Topics included ozone depletion, global warming, and overpopulation. Edward Wilson, a professor from Harvard University and author of *Biophilia,* addressed biodiversity; former Vice President Al Gore presented a lecture on "Ecology and the Human Spirit"; and Carl Sagan (1934-1996), former professor of astronomy at Cornell University, gave the lecture "A Vision of the Future." The conference concluded with a resolution stating that the environment is a gift from God and the

> future of this gift so freely given is in our hands and we must maintain it as we have received it. This is an inescapably reli-

gious challenge. . . . There is a call for moral transformation, as we recognize that the roots of environmental destruction lie in human pride, greed and selfishness, as well as the appeal of the short-term over the long term. We reaffirm here, in the strongest possible terms, the indivisibility of social justice and ecological integrity.[24]

The Harvard University Center for the Study of World Religions released a three-year analysis of the environmental teachings of ten major religions. Center Director Lawrence Sullivan believes that environmentalists have not fully utilized religious perspectives on the relationship between people and the earth. "Change won't happen without religions because they are the touchstone of people's deepest motivations," he was quoted as saying at a news conference at the United Nations.

The National Council of Churches, the nation's largest coalition of Protestant and Orthodox Christian denominations, is in the midst of a campaign to push for national and international action on global warming. In northern California, the Central Conference of American Rabbis, the nation's leading organization of Reform Judaism, teamed up with a local group known as the Redwood Rabbis. The National Religious Partnership for the Environment (NRPE), the nation's largest interfaith coalition, includes member groups such as African-American Protestants, Jews, Catholics, and Eastern Orthodox and evangelical Christians. The Coalition on the Environment and Jewish Life covers global warming, energy policy, environmental health, and biodiversity issues. Tony Campolo, author and a leading evangelist, has written that Christians have turned deaf ears on pleas to save God's creation. In his 1990 World Day of Peace message, Pope John Paul II declared the ecological crisis to be a common responsibility.[25]

Naturally, there is opposition. In 1999, theologians, economists, and environmental experts gathered at a conference center in Connecticut to discuss what they interpreted as religious environmentalism moving in an alarming direction. Environmentalist movements in the 1980s were criticized for maintaining a focus on wetlands and wilderness, and for not expressing enough concern for issues of racism, economic justice, and inadequate health care.[26] With the advent of nonprofit organizations such as Land's Sake and the ecoministry of Evergreen (see Chapter 6), there *is* a prominent shift to address so-

cial issues concurrent with teaching environmental issues. These organizations teach agriculture, donate produce to food banks, and thus
instill a sense of concern for others. These values can be incorporated
into our schools, churches, and other organizations. We can attend
to social problems in the context of environmental and agricultural
programs, as organizations such as Land's Sake and Evergreen make
evident.

As I have previously mentioned, if environmental values are not
instilled at a young age, these attitudes may never develop. An analogy
is found in the separation of the health care and food industries. The
food industry is ignorant of the health care system and the health care
system is ignorant of the food industry. They seem to be mutually exclusive of each other—separate entities. Does it make any sense that
we are feeding patients with foods laden with *trans* fatty acids and
hydrogenated fats while physicians are trying to cure them? There is
an inherent and obvious relationship between health and food, yet we
treat these two factors as independent entities. This is completely il-
logical and irrational. The same principle holds true in the relationship between religion and ecology. And because we fail to acknowledge this relationship, we suffer. If the church restores its ties to
nature, it can be a prominent influence to those seeking solace, particularly those who struggle with learning disabilities. If one seeks a
church as a social support and is renewed through a relationship with
the earth, and hence God, one may derive the same psychological and
social benefits from environmental education that I have previously
mentioned.

Simply start with a garden at your school or church. For information on grants and funding, see Appendix B. Join an environmental
organization or initiate a group in your church, whether for adults or
youths. There are many rivers, lakes, and highways littered with garbage. Many farms offer "gleaning" days when church groups are welcome to harvest produce for homeless shelters and soup kitchens.
This tradition is based on a verse from Scripture, Leviticus 23:22:
"When you harvest your fields, do not cut the grain at the edges of the
fields, and do not go back to cut the heads of grain that were left;
leave them for poor people and foreigners."

Innumerable people in this world have voices and many talents,
with the potential to be great activists, but have no outlets for such expression. Often, they have been suppressed, discouraged, or without

guidance or direction. Churches are one solution to help countless souls nurture their spirituality through a concern for the earth. In turn, this may nourish a relationship with the church and God. Creating an awareness of the relationship between religion and ecology *will* eventually address social concerns, such as emotional and psychological disorders, poverty, and our physical health.

Chapter 6

In the Trenches

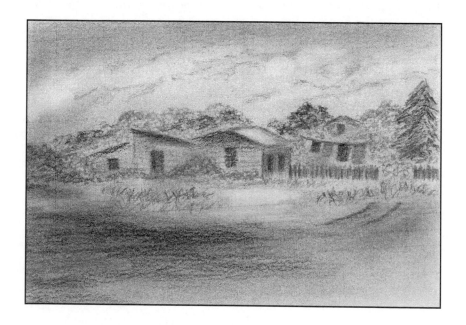

Have you really lived ten thousand or more days, or have you lived one day ten thousand or more times?

Anonymous

My parents and sister are traveling to Farmington, Maine, with our church in early July 1995 to build houses in impoverished communities for an organization called Mission at the Eastward (MATE), similar to Habitat for Humanity. I decide, on a whim, to hop on board at the last minute. We travel in a caravan of minivans and RVs, a group of approximately fifteen kids and fifteen adults, to this little rural community that does not even qualify for a dot on a state map.

As the sun is setting, we pull in the driveway at Stone Hall, where we will be living for the next week. Hordes of people pile out of the vans, stretching weary legs. I lug my suitcase over my shoulder and trudge up to the first floor to check in and get a room key. Five minutes later, I settle in my room with another girl. The room is sparsely furnished, with a bare tile floor, but I imagine I will be grateful for any bed at the end of each day. There is a bathroom across from us, but it is designated for the men. I attempt to cover it up with a "women only" sign, but the men insist it is theirs. Change is inevitable, I try to reason, but I am outnumbered and defeated.

After everyone is situated, we crowd back into the vans and the kids go to a Pizza Hut while the adults opt for lobster. After dinner, we go back to the dorms and then walk through the town to Gifford's for ice cream. Contentedly eating ice cream, we wander over to the central part of town and listen to the Old Crow band play their annual concert, attended by townspeople in cars and on foot. At the conclusion of each song, horns blare in response. The "town" is essentially an old movie theater, a bar, a general store, and a thrift shop. After the concert, we head back to the dorms, where everyone wanders around for a while until we hit the sack.

Seven o'clock comes quickly and loud thumping on my door awakens me. It persists until I wearily drag myself out of bed and answer the door, if only to stop the ceaseless knocking. It is, of course, my mother.

"Breakfast is in ten minutes. If you miss a ride, you're stuck here," she says glaring at me.

"Well, that means I can go back to sleep, right?"

"Ten minutes!"

I close the door, tie my hair back, and rummage through my suitcase that I have neglected to unpack. I scrounge up a T-shirt and pair of cutoffs, throw on some work boots, and am ready to go. Sleep will indisputably take precedence over showering this week.

By 7:30, everyone stumbles out of the dorm and into cars to go to the town church for breakfast. Actually, we eat breakfast in the basement, like moles underground. The sanctuary upstairs is a small room complete with long wooden benches for pews, and the director of MATE welcomes us. An amiable, down-to-earth person, he describes his experiences directing a summer camp, escaping the pressures of contemporary society, leaving behind cell phones, beepers, answering machines, and televisions. Unfortunately, these efficient communication devices are considered by many to be the bare necessities of life.

Society today depends on external, passive sources for entertainment. In *The Unsettling of America,* Wendell Berry summarizes the plight of many Americans, who are trapped in a vicious circle of making money and entertaining themselves:

> He earns money, typically as a specialist, working an eight-hour day at a job for the quality or consequences of which somebody else—or perhaps more typically, nobody else—will be responsible. And not surprisingly, since he can do so little else for himself, he is even unable to entertain himself, for there exists an enormous industry of exorbitantly expensive specialists whose purpose is to entertain him. . . . He feels that all his possessions are under threat of pillage. . . . The household that can provide some of its own pleasures will not be helplessly dependent on the entertainment industry, will influence it by not being helplessly dependent on it, and will not support it thoughtlessly out of boredom.[1]

A classic, spiritually based vocational concern is whether to pursue a career for its monetary rewards or the ability to serve one's community or humanity. The influence of today's materially centered culture causes people to see their careers primarily in financial terms, rather than as outlets for their spiritual need to create a world of love and justice.[2]

After church, we drive into the mountains for a barbecue and to play volleyball. It is a beautiful day; the sun bursts through white, puffy clouds embroidered on an aqua blue sky. We are invited by the landowner to tour an old, historical house nearby that has been converted into a museum honoring Nordica, a famous opera star born in 1857. Mannequins display her custom-made gowns and exquisite costumes. I stand in her bedroom and stare at the hand-knitted white bedspread, trying to imagine the birth of Nordica in this very room.

For the remainder of the afternoon, we tour the work sites for the coming week. The first stop is an old house divided into apartments. Immediately, I notice the peeling and chipped exterior. I have a hunch

I will be assigned here to paint. We climb back into our cars and drive a few miles until we turn onto a narrow, gravel drive. At the top, we reach the Kirschbaums' house, a ramshackle building comprised of a trailer and semifinished addition that requires the completion of a steel roof. The backyard is a tangled mass of overgrown thicket and restless weeds. Laundry hangs sporadically on ropes strung between trees, and several dogs lie in the shade, panting from the July humidity. Two disheveled teenage boys wander down the broken wooden steps, eyeing us suspiciously. An overweight woman in a sleeveless T-shirt and floral shorts follows the boys.

"Hi!" she says enthusiastically. "Welcome! We're so glad you're all here. See what the last group started?" She beckons toward the roof. "The rain don't come in no more. I got real tired of putting them buckets all over. When are you guys coming back?"

"We'll be starting tomorrow, Mrs. Kirschbaum," one of the men from our group says.

"Great! I'll make up a batch of lemonade today."

We say our good-byes in chorus and head to the next site, a one-room shack nestled into the mountainside. A pretty girl with tangled long brown hair opens the door, a young child clinging to her legs. She looks to be no more than twenty-one.

"Hi, we're from MATE, the crew who'll be working on your house," someone announces.

"Hi," she says shyly. "I'm Cara. Do you want to come in and look around?"

"Sure." We file into a tiny area functioning as an all-purpose room for the kitchen and living room. A stove lodged in one corner is piled high with dishes and food, and two frayed couches and a desk line the opposite wall. A wooden frame partitions off one corner for what we are told is to be a bathroom. They presently have no running water or true bathroom, relying on the woods or a neighbor's house down the mountain. The floor consists of bare plywood, and a miniature basement houses a bunk bed for Courtney, the three-year-old wrapped around Cara's leg. Outside, the surrounding area is strewn with broken furniture, weeds, flat tires, rusty bed frames, and the rotting corpse of a truck partially embedded in the soil. Cara's husband is working under the hood of a jalopy, but he pokes his head out when he hears us.

"Hi," he says cheerily. "You the next crew?"

"Yup. We're from New Jersey," someone volunteers.

"I'm Greg." He wipes his oil-stained hands off on a rag and extends one to a few of us.

"How long have you lived here?" someone asks.

"Born and bred in Maine. My father lived up here and I ain't never been anywhere else. Don't want to, neither. So you coming tomorrow?"

"Yeah, some of us will be here first thing in the morning. I understand we'll be working on the bathroom and building a bedroom downstairs?"

"That's right. The last group started the bathroom. Sure'll be nice not to have to truck on down to my neighbor's house. I worry about Cara and all. We're gonna have ourselves another baby and it'll be easier for her."

We discuss the house for a few more minutes, bid our good-byes, and drive back to the dorms for dinner.

Loud banging on the door. Muffled sounds. Groggily, I raise my head. The clock reads 6:30. I pull the sheet over my head and burrow under the pillow. Five more minutes. I open my eyes again and hear people leaving for breakfast. Frantic, I jump out of bed, throw on work clothes, and wash my face. Par for the course, I am the last one but manage to catch the last car departing for the church. The basement is mass chaos as some are eating breakfast while others are packing lunch. Two people from our church volunteer each year to cook for the week, while the remaining folk go to the work sites. Peanut butter and jelly, tuna fish, and egg salad are laid out on the table as we stuff sandwiches together for lunch.

By 8 a.m., we're on our work site. My hunch is correct, and I am placed on High Street, the three-story house converted to apartment buildings, to paint, so everyone is assured I won't nail myself to the wall. I am directed to the huge Victorian porch, along with two other crew members, to scrape and paint. After an hour or so, I find myself almost enjoying the rhythmic scraping and peeling away of old layers, preparing a smooth surface for a fresh coat of paint. It is almost, dare I say, meditative. Soon I am happily immersed in my own world and highly intent on this one project. I am oblivious to the rest of the world, and time escapes me. Nothing exists at this moment but the present, a difficult state of mind to achieve.

As I scrape around the windowsill, I catch fragments of conversation from the people inside. I hear a child and a teenage girl discussing the talk show they are watching. I am an intruder who is privy to these conversations. The girl inside does not acknowledge us, although we have been scraping all morning. By lunchtime, I collapse into a chair and fall asleep. Navajo white paint swims before me, imprinted on my mind. At some point, from the depths of my unconsciousness, I hear the snap of a camera directly in front of me, probably to be posted on a bulletin board at church.

Spirits lift in the afternoon, thanks to the peanut butter and jelly sandwiches. Later, I overhear that the girl watching talk shows is only fifteen, is pregnant, and lives with her boyfriend. The child who was inside watching television with her ventures out and stands in the driveway, intently watching us. She looks to be about twelve or thirteen. My father, amiable as always, approaches her. My father can elicit anyone's life story within the first five minutes of a conversation; it really is an admirable trait. I work up enough courage to introduce myself and ask her a few questions. She happily tells us she is in sixth grade and lives in a trailer down the road. She refuses my father's offer to paint with us but sits on the lawn and watches. I can only interpret this behavior as a sign of some trust, although cautious. She delineates clear boundaries but perches on the perimeter.

At four, we conclude work for the day, and I am exhausted. Just as the fantasy of nestling into my bed for a catnap begins to unfold, we are whisked off to the nearby Sandy River for a swim. I dive into the invigorating water and surface, watching the droplets trickle down my arms and glisten in the late afternoon sun. There is nothing greater than to be alive and reveling in this moment of bliss and contentment. I feel cleansed, renewed, almost as if this were a second baptism. I swim to the other side of the river, climb onto a boulder, and watch the waves lap over the edge of the rocks. I close my eyes and bask in the warming rays of the sun, as droplets of water slowly evaporate from my body. Soon, a voice breaks my concentration: a call from the other side to return to the dorms. I reluctantly climb off the rock and swim back.

Later that night, after dinner, we gather upstairs in the sanctuary for vespers, an informal time of song and worship. My sister strums her guitar while we sing a few songs, then some of us discuss our day. My father broaches the subject of "bridging the gap" and describes our conversations with the residents of High Street. A couple of others relay similar experiences, and we discuss our frustrations, our roles as outsiders. Many things went through my mind over the course of the day. Sometimes I questioned why I was doing this. Did anyone even care?

Someone asks the question I am thinking. "Perhaps we aren't meant to always see results," someone volunteers. "Maybe there is no obvious appreciation, but we may have an impact on their lives that we don't know about."

"There's also the issue of trust, resentment, and cynicism. I'm sure many of these people think we have ulterior motives and are just doing this to relieve our consciences, and we're going to return to our affluent lifestyles," someone else says.

I mull this over for a while. I do feel a sense of accomplishment. I believe we made a difference in someone's life, done selflessly or not. I do not believe pure altruism exists; everyone stands to gain something. We all have our reasons for coming to Maine, and we derive personal benefits from these experiences, whether to justify our lifestyles, relieve our consciences, or seek fulfillment in our lives where there are voids. I cannot shake the feelings of guilt I have; this is natural. But I think we must accept our fates and live together on earth, trying to improve one another's lives. Humans are created equally, but we exist in a capitalistic society where money is not dispersed equally. One should not feel guilt, but appreciate and savor good fortune and try to change the world instead of simply feeling pity for those less fortunate. My question on apathy is addressed the next day. I change my mind the next day while we are painting. A tenant walks over, smiles briefly, and nods. "Nice job," he says and walks into his apartment. Later in the day, we meet Jamie and her son Mike. A group worked on her house a couple years ago, as she received welfare. Today, she is employed full-time as a nurse and runs a small thrift shop. When our church returns each year, she and Mike work with us for the week and participate in all the activities. She gives back what she received, and I believe she is symbolic of many others we don't see. Her gratefulness and appreciation overwhelm me. I knew then it was never for nothing; the rewards were far greater.

That night at vespers, the Kirschbaums join us. Another crew is completing the steel roof and building an addition on their trailer. During the closing prayer, Mr. Kirschbaum, who is physically disabled, spoke quietly: "Thank you God, for these wonderful people who have come to help us." I did not question anymore if we made a difference.

By Thursday, it is close to 100 degrees in the shade. We have started working on a new site in the town of Jay, nearly forty minutes away from Farmington. This particular house needs all the window trim painted, a new porch floor, and the entire porch scraped and painted. Irma, an elderly woman, resides here, and she is hooked up to an oxygen tank because of emphysema. There are warning signs banning smoking plastered on the door. I am aghast to discover her puffing away on cigarettes. I pray the house will not spontaneously combust while we are there. I glance around. The house itself is neat and orderly and is luxurious compared to the Kirschbaums. My perspective has changed overnight. "Luxuries" are now a bathroom, telephone, and running water. I am surprised to see paintings hanging on every wall. I walk over to some paintings of landscapes she has framed and hung on the walls. They are signed by the same artist. Why am I surprised? I have to be honest; I didn't expect to see paintings. Life is filled with lessons.

"Who is the artist?" I ask politely.

"My daughter!" she exclaims in a raspy voice.

"How long has she painted?"

"Well, she's always painted. She entered some contest and won first place. She's got a lot of talent, that girl. Gets it from my side," she says proudly.

"Do you paint?"

"Nah, wish I could, but it's not one of the gifts God's chosen to give to me. My daddy painted, that's where she gets it from."

"I hope she keeps painting. They're beautiful."

"Thank you, dear. Now speaking of painting, you kind folks are here to paint this ratty old porch I got here? Be careful of the bees; there's a bunch of angry ones that chased the last group out of here."

"Oh! Well, thanks for the advice. We'll be careful."

We spend the better part of the afternoon scraping. After lunch, I collapse onto a blanket under a tree and fall asleep for an hour. I transform into a wet rag in the humidity, but everyone is tired and breaks periodically throughout the afternoon. Inevitably, we disturb the bee nest, and they angrily swarm around our heads, stinging my father twice.

His hand swells to balloon proportions and he quits for the day, soaking his hand in ice.

Thursday night brings respite for everyone. We journey to Smalls Falls, beautiful, massive waterfalls cascading down the mountains. We hike up the mountain and the adventurous ones jump off the cliffs into the falls, while the rest of us swim in the water below. After an hour, we hike down to a barbecue prepared by two women from church. Someone lights a campfire when the sun sets, and we huddle around the burning embers. The pungent odor of charred pine wafts from the fire, and I inhale deeply. I snuggle into my jacket, warm and content. My parents sit next to me, and my sister plays guitar, leading us in song. I close my eyes and listen to the rush and gurgling of the waterfalls and the crackling of the fire. I want to record the sound and bring it home, but I will have to listen from memory.

I am delirious to be isolated in a world devoid of communication: no telephones, television, computers, answering machines, or mail. Few people understand that we once lived without these "necessities." During this week, we have focused solely on our mission: to refurbish houses. The world would benefit if more people escaped from the chaos and tangle of communication, caught up in the daily grind of meetings, faxes, and phone calls. In *Dream of the Earth,* Thomas Berry writes, "Our difficulty is that we are just emerging from a technological entrancement . . . during this period the human mind has been placed within the narrowest confines it has experienced since consciousness emerged from its Paleolithic phase."[3]

Popular psychotherapy deals primarily with the alienation that exists in contemporary society, and technology dominates much of our daily lives.[4] Although technology has provided us with opportunities and many advantages, it has cost us relationships with one another and the environment. Recently, on a train, I was appalled by the number of people speaking loudly on their cell phones and counted three cell phones in the surrounding seats. Can we not exist in silence anymore or exchange pleasantries with other passengers? Gone forever will be the days of dinners with family and friends, once an opportune time for social discourse and exchange of ideas. Technology often serves as a means to an end. The emphasis in the workforce is quantity and speed, regardless of sacrifices in the spheres of health, social and family obligations, and the environment. Does technology really serve us or are we serving technology?

David Ehrenfeld, an ecology professor at Rutgers University and author of *Beginning Again: People and Nature in the New Millennium,* describes the formidable task of competing for the attention of his students:

> My students have been watching and listening in some cases for five hours a day or more, starting at age two or three. I cannot compete. . . . [T]heir authority figures are two-dimensional and cannot hear. They neither take offense nor do they rebuke; their brief utterances are well suited to the wandering, superficial mentality fostered by the ever-flickering tube. The world of television, by inducing passivity and unresponsiveness, has cut many of the human threads and connections that once bound people together into working communities.[5]

Ehrenfeld refers to contemporary society as "electronically linked" through television, the Internet, e-mail, and voice mail, inducing passivity and alienation far from the virtues of community. He laments that almost every technological advance brings more social disintegration.

Roszak and colleagues state:

> People experience deep pleasure and release from sweating together, feeling the elements of soil and water, rock and plant, while doing a common task with a visible positive outcome. Living as part of an earthy, purposeful community becomes intensely tangible. Many people who usually work in isolation form spontaneous little teams; when doing restoration, people become involved with a place in a very active and embodied manner.[6]

Margaret Mead postulated that people's self-images depend in large part on their social images, as reflected in the eyes of others in their social groups. When people substitute a new society for their former one, their self-images are likely to change as well.

The next day, we finish what is possible. We beg, plead, and cajole our crew chief into leaving by two. The heat is stifling. Someone has mixed acrylic and oil paint together and we are unable to finish the porch. Two days of work remain, but the next group will resume where we left off.

We say good-bye to Irma. She seems lonely and is quite talkative, although she huffs and puffs without the assistance of her oxygen. She wishes us an enjoyable summer, and I wonder how much longer she will be around. It would have been nice to work with a family for a week, as we really did not have the opportunity to "bond" with anyone. However, it is intriguing to catch small glimpses into other people's lives.

We swim once more in the Sandy River, and I am sad to be leaving the next day. New Jersey pales in comparison to the beauty of New England. This experience has offered me the seclusion, serenity, camaraderie, and companionship with a select group of people I cared very deeply for by the end of the week.

Community service is therapeutic and builds community; indisputably, it should be included in general and alternative educational curricula. Installing community service projects within a curricula may eventually improve cooperation within classrooms. When students, or others, work together on a shared task in the context of a community, an appreciation for others' talents and respect for one another develop. Community service experiences are an invaluable tool that far surpasses group therapy for adolescents. These experiences teach values such as caring for others. Empathy develops when one becomes aware of the plight and suffering of others and stops dwelling on one's own problems. This also gives one an internal locus of control, the belief that one has the ability to change things in the world, instead of playing a passive role in life, influenced by forces beyond one's control. Accordingly, optimism may develop that replaces a pessimistic view of life, and that optimism comes with a sense of spiritual fulfillment or reward from helping someone else who suffers. Self-esteem and confidence develop as one helps others. Within the context of a group experience, barriers are broken down and communication improves, as a task becomes a group effort. Community service projects require a variety of gifts that people from all walks of life can offer. People often discover traits and qualities about themselves that may even encourage other career or avocational pursuits, such as joining the Peace Corps, becoming a social worker, or working on environmental campaigns to improve water quality in third-world countries.

A study of thirty adolescents ranging in age from nine to seventeen years participated in a project called Project Back-on-Track (BOT), a multimodal after-school program designed to act as an early intervention to prevent youths from committing future criminal offenses. The adolescents represented a diverse ethnic group of 63.3 percent African Americans, 33.3 percent Caucasians, and 3.3 percent Hispanics. The majority of the youths, 93 percent, had at least one current DSM-IV diagnosis, including conduct disorder (63.3 percent), ADHD (23.3 percent), dysthymia (23.3 percent), major depressive episode (16.7 percent), marijuana abuse/dependence (10 percent), and alcohol abuse/dependence (6.7 percent). During BOT, no psychopharmacological treatment was administered.[7]

Participants in the BOT program met for two hours every day after school, four days a week, for a duration of four weeks. Staff and participants jointly selected two-hour community service projects that encouraged empathy for others and contributed to the community. During the one-year follow-up study, the community control group committed eighteen more crimes than the BOT group. The program reaped economic benefits and demonstrated a savings of $1,800 per youth at one year after BOT participation. Therefore, it may be stated that community service-based programs can contribute economic, social, and psychological benefits to society. Furthermore, they may serve as an early intervention to prevent future criminal offenses and perhaps even diminish the likelihood of chronic adult psychological or psychiatric disorders.

Mexico

About thirty of us are sequestered on the roof of the sanctuary. Although it is about 1 a.m., Mexican music reverberates through the night and a group of men are sitting on stools in front of a house across the street, slugging down tequila. Deep, booming laughter punctuates their conversation, while stray roosters crow and an occasional horse-drawn buggy clops down the dirt road. Inside, the sanctuary is a stifling 120 degrees, thus the reason we have retreated to the roof to sleep, which now is a sea of sleeping bags. I settle into my sleeping bag, trying to find a comfortable way to lie on the concrete underneath me. There is none. Sweaty and exhausted, I climb off the roof at one point to sleep for a while in one of our rental vans. Other leaders and kids are stretched out in the seats so I settle into a vacant one. Soon, a mosquito buzzes around my ear, and no matter how many times I swat at the air, it returns. I pull my sleeping bag over my face, but it is suffocating. I give up and return to the roof. I drift in and out of consciousness the rest of the night, finally waking up stiff and groggy in the morning to a warm, humid breeze. I wipe the excess oil from my face, rake my fingers through my coarse, dry hair, and shake out my damp sleeping bag covered with dust. Most of the kids have already climbed down to wait in line for one of two bathrooms.

Somehow sixty people manage to dress and look presentable for a church service led by two local ministers in the one-room sanctuary. Most of it is spoken and sung in Spanish, and I muddle through. My Spanish is rusty, although I can comprehend enough. Hymnals are few and far between. A woman standing next to me taps me on the arm and shares her book with me. After the service, we caravan in vans to the dormitory where we will reside for the following week. The temperature has already climbed well above 100 degrees, and I watch the scenery speed by, as I relax comfortably in the air-conditioned van, sheltered from the dust. Guilt strikes as we amble past ramshackle houses, comprised of miscellaneous pieces of wood and tin tacked together. Scantily clothed children wander in the street, horses pull wagons laden with garbage, and groups of men congregated on corners outside of grocery stores scrutinize us.

We turn onto a bumpy, dirt road and park next to a two-story building comprised of gray cinder blocks. The second story is partially finished; there is no roof and most of the "windows" are nothing more than openings. A wrought iron gate fence surrounds the compound, lending it the look of a fortress. I frantically look around for another building, perhaps across the street, where we will reside. Perhaps, we are stopping here only temporarily. Someone opens the van doors and kids and suitcases topple out. I follow with the sinking feeling that we will not be going anywhere anytime soon. I drag my suitcase out onto the dirt floor in the open courtyard.

"Boys on the left, girls on the right," Craig directs. The one big open room resembles an orphanage, filled with rows of bunk beds on a concrete slab floor. A floor fan rests on a roll-away bed in the front, and I throw my suitcase on top to claim it.

"Hey, no fair," my sister whines.

"Tough. I've paid my dues," I retort.

She grudgingly walks away and throws her suitcase on a bunk. Around my bed, on either side, are two bathrooms with two toilets and two shower stalls. A distinct stench wafts from the bathroom.

Craig yells into the room, "Meeting in five minutes in the court-yard!"

I change my clothes but soon discover it is senseless as they are coated in a permanent layer of dust. I wander out into the courtyard where leaders and kids are mingling. Bryce, the coordinator of the organization, Puentes de Cristo, explains that the plumbing rarely functions so we cannot flush any toilet paper down the toilets. It must be disposed of in wastebaskets. I grimace at the thought of the odor by the end of the week, although it will be taken out daily. He further explains that running water is scarce and showers are rare. We must fill up a big tin of water, lug it into the shower, and pour cups of water over ourselves.

Meals will be done in shifts. Two Mexican women will prepare lunch every day, but we will set out breakfast and cook dinner in groups. Breakfast is at 8, and we leave for work sites at 8:30. Those not on work sites in the morning will teach vacation Bible school. We spend the rest of the day lounging around the courtyard, playing cards, reading, and walking to the corner grocery for soda. I talk to Bryce for a while, sitting against an outside railing on the second-floor walkway. His room is about eight by ten feet with one bunk bed and a pole that extends across for hanging his clothes. He has lived here for a year and is battling with the town to improve the water quality. Many households do not have running water, and, if they do, it is not drinkable. Women and children lug buckets of water from wells, or those who can afford it buy water from a local store. His dedication and commitment are admirable, having left his family and friends to live in a foreign, impoverished land.

While we are talking, the sky turns shades of lilac and, soon, little is visible. Night falls quickly, and the kids are rowdy, off in groups talking and giggling. Bryce needs to talk to Craig before he goes to sleep, and I walk over to another section of the building, the area without any roof. Some of our group will be constructing the roof this week. I find an opening that serves as a window and perch myself on the ledge. The stars are blurry, clouded by the thick, damp air. I watch three teenage boys on the street below steal a vendor's cart, laughing and speaking in fragmented Spanish. I wonder what their purpose is. Is it only mischief? I pity the poor, hardworking vendor who will be shocked the next morning to discover his livelihood gone. On the next block, Mexican music emanates from a small shack and laughter rings through the night. For all the poverty, abundant joy is prevalent everywhere, at least present in the form of music. Everyone seems happy. Many Americans are miserable, selling their souls to corporations in exchange for the purpose of attaining innumerable possessions. Take away the possessions and what do you have? These people had few, if any, possessions, but joy—mixed with an expression of placidity—was etched into their faces. I glance down to the ground and wonder how it would feel to fly. I have this sudden, scary urge to jump, and it frightens me that this random thought has popped into my mind.

Suddenly, I sense that I am not alone, and I look over at another window. A figure is curled up on the ledge, gazing out into the night. I distinctly recognize the features of Catie, one of my sister's friends. I jump down off the ledge and quietly stroll over.

"I see you have the same idea," I say quietly.

"I needed some space. Know what I mean?" she says.

"Yeah, I do. Needed some space, myself. It's been a rough couple of days, huh?"

She nods, and then looks out at the horizon.

"Do you ever wonder what it'd be like to fly?" she says suddenly.

Startled, I look at her. I nod. "Yeah, I do. Funny you should mention that."

"Do you think it would even matter? Life sucks, anyway, then you die. What's the point?"

"Well, Catie, I have to be honest. I feel the same way sometimes."

It is her turn to look startled. "You do?"

"Yeah! But I think many people feel that way at one time or another. Life is tough and I sure fight my share of battles. But you need to have faith, even if it's difficult during many times, but that faith serves a higher purpose. There's something more to this life, but in the meantime, we need to derive as much joy from it as possible. I do understand how you feel, believe me. I had a really tough time growing up, and I think I'm pretty fortunate to have turned out how I did, which isn't so bad." I smile.

She reverts back to gazing out into the night and some time elapses before either of us speaks. She sniffles, and I watch a tear trickle down her cheek. I have known Catie for many years, and she is a younger version of myself, angry and confused. She brings tears to my eyes as she hugs me.

"I love you, Amy."

"I love you, too, Catie. You're going to make me cry," I scold softly. I don't know why I struggle so hard to repress tears.

"You'll be okay, I promise. If I turned out okay, so will you." We talk for a few more minutes, and then I say goodnight and head downstairs for bed.

It is about ninety degrees by 8:30 a.m. as we trudge toward the work sites. My group is spackling and painting the outside of a church. Our foreman, Juan, tells us that he works on the construction site all day and then works second shift in one of the American factories to support his wife and four children. We determine that he earns the equivalent of five American dollars per day. Amazingly, he is good-natured as well as energetic, contrary to many Americans who meld with their couch cushions after an eight-hour day.

Next to the church, a health clinic offers checkups, nutrition classes, and free lunches every day for children. A nurse explains that this is often the only meal of the day for many of them. I remember fasting once for twenty-four hours for a fund-raiser, but I knew it was only temporary, and, once the time period concluded, I knew where to find a refrigerator stocked with anything I desired. On one wall, a rack holds toothbrushes as far as the eye can see. Most of the children do not have access to a sanitary water supply and brush their teeth here.

We spackle and paint for the entire day, breaking only for water and lunch back at the compound. Sweat trickles down my back, and I finally accept the fact that I won't feel clean for quite a while.

Toward the end of the day, we are invited to a church service that night inside the sanctuary. It is satisfying to spend some time inside after kneeling on the ground to spackle a wall. Several Mexican women pass out soda as we arrange ourselves in a circle of folding chairs on the concrete floor. Although I can speak and comprehend basic Spanish, most of the youth group cannot. However, the language barrier does not preclude us from singing songs, both in Spanish and English. Finally, we conclude and walk back to the compound, where I take my bucket shower. The water is cold, but I do not want anything even remotely lukewarm. I use a plastic cup to pour the water over my head when I finish shampooing my hair. I feel clean momentarily, but once I step out, the dampness curls my hair and clings to my skin.

We eat dinner from paper plates while sitting on benches in the courtyard. Faces bear differing degrees of redness, but everyone shares exhaustion. However, we still manage to stay up late, playing cards on the roof. I periodically glance up to watch the stars twinkle down at me. During the week, we settle into a routine: work all day, stay up late at night playing cards and giggling. Montezuma's revenge strikes my sister and a few others one night. She turns green and sequesters herself in the bathroom for hours.

By the end of the week, I am ready for a change in scenery and spend a couple mornings at vacation Bible school. I assist with the arts and crafts, making collages with twenty different children every hour for three classes. The children are adorable, and I marvel at how many look after their younger siblings, already adopting parental roles at the tender ages of seven and eight. I speak to some in broken Spanish and am shocked to discover some do not even attend school but instead work in fast-food restaurants and factories. They appear to be children but wear the weary expressions of grown-ups.

During snack time, they cluster around us like we are a magnetic force attracting them. They grovel for more graham crackers after every box is emptied. The disappointment on their faces makes me want to run to the store and buy hundreds of boxes. At noon, we drive back to the compound for a lunch of homemade tortillas, beans, and rice. We are leaving tomorrow, and I am very excited at the prospect of once again inhaling the scent of grass and trees. Reynosa is a monotone of white dust. However, I cherish the experience and the opportunity to immerse myself in the culture. We are fortunate to have been accepted by the townspeople, despite a few, random cries of "Hey, gringo!" The week ends with small-group discussions of our individual experiences. Many express their fulfillment from working with the kids and are grateful for the opportunity to cross cultural barriers. Others are happy to see the results of the construction on the building and their ability to contribute the necessary labor. We end with a silent, candlelight ceremony, sitting on concrete blocks in the dusty courtyard, a slight breeze rustling the leaves on a nearby tree that has persistently sprung up in the midst of the courtyard.

The next morning is, as always, a flurry of cleaning, packing, and chatter. The layover in Texas is hot and steamy, but we are stationed there for only an hour. The flight home is lengthy, and everyone falls into slumber, fitful though it is on an airplane. Once home, I run barefoot through the grass, crushing the cool blades beneath my feet. I suppress the urge to throw toilet paper in the wastebasket, brush my teeth from a cup, and fill up a tin of water before getting in the shower. I no longer take resources for granted and preserve water, as well as electricity.

* * *

Contrary to popular belief, homelessness and diminished resources are not only a third-world or urban problem. In rural Pennsylvania, where I live, 21,700 people received homeless assistance due to abusive relationships, migrant/seasonal work, and prolonged substance abuse. Statewide, in 1999, nearly 116,000 people received homeless assistance in the forms of rental subsidy, welfare payments, case management, bridge housing (housing and case management service for homeless individuals and families for up to one year), and emergency shelters. According to the Department of Public Welfare, homelessness affects every rural county in Pennsylvania. Unfortunately, resources are limited. According to the the Center for Rural Pennsylvania, almost three times as many people are turned away in rural areas than in urban areas because of a lack of funding on a per capita basis. Many rural homeless are not classified under the urban definition of homelessness, which is sleeping in a shelter or on the street. Many of the rural homeless seek shelter in automobiles or with relatives in overcrowded or inferior housing.[8]

Schools, churches, and community organizations can assist on the local level through food drives during the year (not just holidays), donating produce from gardens, or simply volunteering time to work on repairs needed at the shelter. Before Christmas at our school, we collected food from students and staff to take to a local homeless shelter in Quakertown, Pennsylvania. We sat around a dining-room table while Annette, a social worker and manager, talked to the students about her role as a social worker, the daily life of the residents at the homeless shelter, and the services they provided to the residents, such as job skills training. She led us on a tour around the shelter, explaining the various projects that volunteers from the community and churches worked on, such as painting, organizing food donations, and house repairs. The students listened with interest, and we made plans to return to paint the kitchen.

On our next visit, my co-workers, Stephanie and Matt, and a handful of students and I painted the large, Victorian kitchen. Initially, I was hesitant about the enthusiasm they would muster, but, within five minutes, students covered all the surface counters and floors with drop cloths and stood on counters, paintbrushes quickly smearing coats of white paint over the nicked and soiled walls. Despite conflicts that emerged on occasion in class, they cooperated with one another and covered the walls in less than two hours, including all the molding. Annette snapped pictures of us, and when she recently visited our school, she presented us with a framed collage, a gift commemorating a memorable afternoon.

Farming is also community service and can play a role in assisting food banks and homeless shelters. According to the *Farmland Preservation Report's Sixth Annual Survey,* four Pennsylvania counties, Lancaster, Chester, York, and Berks, are among the top twelve counties in the nation preserving local farmland.[9] And it is such farmland preservation programs that inevitably contribute to solutions for the social problem of homelessness. Some organizations, such as Land's Sake (see Chapter 3), donate produce from their gardens and farms to food banks. Brian Donahue, a founder, developed a program that teaches farming to suburban middle school children. Not only does the program instill farming, business, and marketing skills, but it also cultivates a value system through its community efforts and exemplary role models. Land's Sake donates organic produce to homeless shelters and food banks in Boston, where students cook and serve meals. At the end of September each year, Land's Sake holds Harvest for Hunger. Dozens of volunteers from the surrounding town of Weston help harvest the bulk of squash and potatoes and send thousands of pounds of vegetables to Boston food banks. Children and adults can also be sponsored during a "pick-a-thon" to help defray the cost of growing food. Similar to the concept of a walk-a-thon, a pick-a-thon involves a few cents donated for every pound of squash or potatoes that are loaded into burlap bags and carried to the edge of the field. In social work, this may be viewed as a systems perspective, as interactive relationships are cultivated among community members and outside organizations.

Land's Sake also encourages land stewardship, a virtue that should be emphasized in all environmental and general educational curricula. A steward is one who manages an institution, a farm, a sport, or the domestic concerns of family life. In *The Gift of Good Land,* Wendell Berry discusses the Christian notion of stewardship: God has given the earth to us as a gift, and we are stewards of the land. A verse from Scripture supports this view: "They will certainly build houses and have occupancy; and they will certainly plant vineyards and eat their fruitage" (Isaiah 65:21-22). Stewardship teaches one a sense of responsibility and respect for the earth, not domination or destruction. Stewardship involves practicing sustainability and using what one needs with respect for nonrenewable natural resources. I believe this concept can also be generalized to the self and, in particular, to people struggling with self-destructive behaviors, such as addiction.

A recent article in *Organic Gardening,* a Rodale Institute publication, describes the ecoministry of Evergreen, a 728-acre farm in western Pennsylvania that is home to the Sisters of the Humility of Mary. After hearing a calling to tend the earth, Sister Barbara O'Donnell determinedly initiated a farming program with the help of Frank Romeo, a caretaker. Despite sluggish profits and a decline of women entering religious life, Sister Barbara worked with Romeo to develop three acres of organic gardens. About 80 percent of the organic produce, with a market value of approximately $25,000, is donated to the poor. The community's kitchen and cafeteria uses the remaining food to feed the 100 sisters in residence, as well as other staff who work there during the day. In addition, Evergreen offers workshops on solar energy, alternative healing, organic cooking, world hunger, and simple living.[10]

Stewardship builds community as well, and, conversely, community builds stewardship. Community-supported agriculture (CSA) programs teach one stewardship in the context of community as well as learning together. CSA originated in Europe and Japan. In Japan, CSA programs are called *teikei,* which translates into "putting the farmer's face on food." CSAs have grown from one in 1986 to more than 600 today.[11] A CSA is a mutual arrangement between local farmers and the community that is cost efficient; transportation costs are reduced as there is no need for distribution. The farmer is granted extra time to tend to his crops because he or she does not need to expend excessive time and energy preparing for markets or selling to restaurants. The extra time also allows for farmers to build relationships with their customers, and many CSAs provide educational workshops to the community and internship programs (see Appendix B). Many members often volunteer time to help harvest, plant, and cultivate crops, as well. It is also an alternative for many small-scale organic farmers who can no longer afford to compete with conventional farmers, as well as a way to preserve farmland. In a CSA, customers buy shares; prices typically begin at $200 per person to $760 for families at the beginning of a season, and they then receive a weekly share of the harvest during the growing season, from May to November.

I recently visited Sam Cantrell's CSA, named Maysie's Farm, in Glenmoore, Pennsylvania. Cantrell is the farm's only full-time employee and has saved his family's sixty-four-acre farm from the clutches of encroaching developers. According to the state's Department of Agriculture, Pennsylvania has lost more than 400,000 acres of farmland between 1991 and 1996.[12] Cantrell provides educational workshops to community and school groups, full moon potluck suppers, community lecture series on a range of agriculture topics, and housing interns each summer, providing them with a stipend and organic food from the six acres of gardens. The internship program, offered throughout the year, is an educational experience that teaches anyone interested in agriculture about sustainability, conservation, and ecological resource management. Interns learn about organic vegetable production and participate in all phases of planning, marketing, and financial management of a CSA. Cantrell also provides educational field trips to other farms so that interns have the opportunity to observe a variety of agricultural practices.

If community members and youths are educated about agriculture through CSA programs and agriculture curricula in schools, farmland preservation programs will continue to increase, making great social contributions and playing a role in the solution to homelessness and hunger. Schools, churches, and other community organizations can introduce mission trips and local mission work efforts into their curricula and agendas. Once again, this gives people a sense of purpose, belonging, and accomplishment, and, often, it introduces new vocational pursuits that may alleviate social and psychological problems such as crime, depression, and poor self-esteem. I can almost guarantee that children and adults with excessive energy will find outlets in community service projects.

Walt, a local farmer, and his wife, Jane, a nurse practitioner, have started a nonprofit Center for Sustainable Living on their farm. During the summer, they offer high school students the opportunity to work on the farm for an hourly wage and participate in two weekly workshops taught by local writers, artists, and photographers. Deb, a local creative writing teacher, and Jen, a local artist, devoted their summer to teaching and directing the program along with Walt and Jane. Throughout the summer, students developed a scrapbook chronicling their experiences on the farm, based on a theme of compassion as found in community, nature, or self. Ultimately, they are instilling values of community, sustainability, and respect for the environment. These students will gain an understanding of local culture and the relationship between farmers and the community. They will comprehend the elements of community and will far surpass many of their peers.

Community service in its simplest definition means providing a service to the community. This service can assume the form of agriculture, building houses for those underserved, or volunteering at a homeless shelter or in a hospital. Essentially, it is anything that builds relationships within the community, but, more than that, the symbiotic relationship between the land and people, a sense of belongingness, rootedness, and a sense of purpose become evident. If we fail to instill the values of community, then inevitably we create a society of drifters, of people without roots and purpose. We create those who follow others lacking a purpose, and this is one of the reasons rampant drug and alcohol problems exist today, along with a plethora of psychological disorders.

Chapter 7

The Silence of the Woods

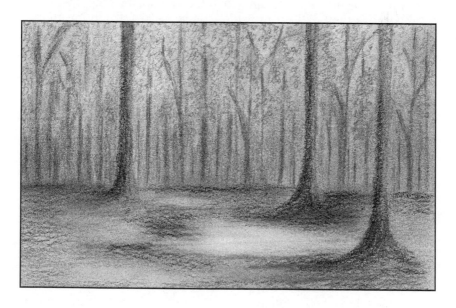

To go in the dark with a light is to know the light.
To know the dark, go dark. Go without sight,
and find that the dark, too, blooms and sings,
and is traveled by dark feet and dark wings.

Wendell Berry

After I leave California, I find a job as a counselor in a Christian camp. We sleep in platform tents in a forest next to a creek, and the gurgling waters lull me to sleep. Nighttime is devoted to campfires, and it is then that the opportunity arises for me to lead a discussion. I nervously crouch on the log and glance around at the faces shadowed in the light of the fire.

"I want to read the Parable of the Sower, one of my favorite passages from Luke, to you," I begin.

> While a large crowd was gathering and people were coming to Jesus from town after town, he told this parable: "A farmer went out to sow his seed. As he was scattering the seed, some fell along the path; it was trampled on, and the birds of the air ate it up. Some fell on rock, and when it came up, the plants withered because they had no moisture. Other seed fell among thorns, which grew up with it and choked the plants. Still other seed fell on good soil. It came up and yielded a crop, a hundred times more than was sown. When he said this, he called out, he who has ears to hear, let him hear. His disciples asked him what this parable meant. He said, the knowledge of the secrets of the kingdom of God has been given to you, but to others I speak in parables, so that, though seeing, they may not see; though hearing, they may not understand. This is the meaning of the parable: The seed is the word of God. Those along the path are the ones who hear, and then the devil comes and takes away the word from their hearts, so that they may not believe and be saved. Those on the rock are the ones who receive the word with joy when they hear it, but they have no roots. They believe for a while, but in the time of testing they fall away. The seed that fell among thorns stands for those who hear, but as they go on their way they are choked by life's worries, riches, and pleasures, and they do not mature. But the seed on good soil stands for those with a noble and good heart, who hear the word, retain it, and by persevering produce a crop." (Luke 8:4-15)

I close my Bible. "Now for the next five minutes, go find a spot, by yourself and just listen to the night, to the silence." A nervous laughter echoes throughout the crowd, but slowly the kids and other counselors disperse. I hear a couple snickers, but within a few minutes, the voices are silent, and thirty or so people are scattered throughout the woods. The moon beams down upon us through the tops of the trees, and I quietly tiptoe through the woods, the dry twigs snapping underneath my feet, and find a spot near the rapids. I crouch down on the ground and gaze into the darkness, closing my eyes. Tranquility settles upon me, and I feel a sense of myself merging with the surrounding environment, a oneness. I listen to the water rushing over the rapids and the stillness of the night, the serenity. Reluctantly, I tear myself away and return to the campfire, calling the others back.

"How many people liked this exercise?"

They all raise their hands.

"What did you experience during this time?" I ask.

One kid raises his hand. "It was really peaceful. I liked it."

A girl raises her hand. "It gave me the chance to think about some things that I usually can't."

"How many of you get an opportunity like this at home to spend a minimum of five minutes in silent contemplation?" No one raises a hand, and I would be surprised if anyone did, including myself. I nod. "Most of us are so busy with school, homework, and work that we don't have the opportunity to pray, talk to God, to nurture our faith. And it's during a time of reflection that we can listen to God; perhaps hear an answer that we've been seeking. Take time in your day to stop and listen to God. Tell Him about your troubles . . . even if it's only five minutes a day. That five minutes can make enough of an impact to significantly change your life for the better." It was a powerful exercise in silence that hopefully prompted the awakening of dulled senses. One may allow thoughts to process that may normally be disrupted by excessive stimuli we encounter in our daily lives.

Later, on the way back to the cabin, I walk with Staffan, who is from Sweden. His unruly, dark shoulder-length hair captivates me, and I admire his ruggedness and casualness, although it is not a reflection of apathy. We discuss our interests in wilderness medicine, and he entertains me with stories of Sweden.

"Turn your flashlight off," he says suddenly.

"Why?" I ask, startled.

"Because. How are you going to learn to rely on your senses?"

"Do you always walk without a flashlight?"

"Yes, because I only need to rely on my senses. You need to train them, sharpen them. You'll be surprised how weak they are now, but how strong they can become."

"Watch," he says.

I turn my flashlight off and at first am terrified. I don't know if I'm about to trip over rocks or walk straight into a tree.

"Just try it for a while," he gently commands. "Your eyes will adjust."

He is right. After five minutes, I can discern the shadows in front of me and the pale light of the moon illuminates the path. And I hear. I am keenly aware of the wind rustling through the trees, chirping crickets, and squirrels scurrying in the nearby bush. Surprisingly, I do not stumble into a tree, and I relax, relinquishing my fears. The overall effect is analogous, ironically, to someone removing a blindfold. My fear dissipates, and I then realize most of us do not progress forward in life unless we feel certainty, and it is only fear that precludes us from venturing into the unknown. We must have light to illuminate the obstacles, every detail, to avoid tripping and falling flat on our faces. However, by squelching that fear and taking risk, we may discover a heightening of our senses and perhaps stumble upon new paths. After that night, I abandon my flashlight.

*   *   *

Zazen, the sitting meditation in the Zen Buddhist tradition, requires one to attend to the present moment. During one class, I was intently focused on waves lapping around the edge of a rock, visualizing my favorite spot on a particular lake. Suddenly, I experienced a sensation of detachment from my body. I was so still; never have I been so still. When Dr. Khalsa, the meditation teacher, finally spoke and rang the bell, his voice was distant. I gradually returned, and there was a definitive period when my mind and body remerged. Almost irritated, I did not want to return. Perhaps this is analogous to the peace of a near-death experience. It is similar to the high of marijuana, but that is a quick, fast fix. This took practice, control, and patience I had not achieved in prior meditation sessions. Ninety minutes passed to my astonishment. Dr. Khalsa delivered an excellent, but brief lecture. He spoke of the phenomena and events in our lives that pull us in a multitude of directions. He spoke of a poet who once said, "Turn your head and there is your life." How reminiscent of my tangential life. A Zen Buddhist stated that distraction is due to a lack of concentration. Hence, if one with ADD/ADHD can discipline the self to meditate, concentration will increase, and this will alleviate the major problem of distraction that many of us encounter. I refer to the simple distraction of noise in our daily lives, as well as the distractions from others who attempt to pull us in a number of directions. When I walked home that evening after meditation, I was conscious of my feet hitting the pavement, the noise it generated as well as the physical sensation. I moved slowly and quietly, feeling quite peaceful, and later settled into a quiet evening of Miles Davis, candles, and reading.

During another meditation class, we chanted in Sanskrit cued by the instructor. This is a Hindu technique of repeatedly chanting a mantra, a sacred thought or prayer. Maharishi Mahesh Yogi first brought transcendental meditation (TM) to the United States in the 1960s. In TM, an instructor selects a mantra, a particular Sanskrit word or sound, for each student (although the instructor often leads a group mantra and does not assign an individual one). The sound is repeated while silently sitting, which discourages distracting thoughts. Physiological changes include a lowered heart rate, decreased blood pressure, and a lowered rate of oxygen consumption.[1]

The candles around the room cast leaping shadows on the walls and the scent of sandalwood drifted from an incense holder. Typically, I need to focus on a visual image (symbolic meditation) and have never fully embraced the idea of chanting. However, feeling quite relaxed from the previous yoga class, my voice suddenly sounded distant, an almost disembodied quality. I swam backward through my mind, parting dark layer after dark layer, traversing the inner depths of my soul. On one level, I was acutely aware of my excitement about returning to this state, but on another level, I continued to pursue a focus on this inward journey. Once again, I experienced a gradual detachment from my physical body but retained my cognitive awareness of it.

On this journey, I thought back to a recent camping trip in Maine where I spent the first evening watching the sun set over a lagoon. I sat on a large, gray boulder, the sand cool and gritty beneath me. The Maine wind gently whistled around me, teasing and toying with the strands of my hair. Scents of nearby bayberry and rosehips wafted through the air, tingling my nostrils. I grasped my knees to my chest and watched the sun descend, a glowing, fiery ball surrounded by flaming streaks of rose-tinted clouds. Gentle waves in the lagoon below lapped around massive boulders. Only my inner tranquility and bliss existed, replacing the apathy I had felt earlier in the day. I stayed on that boulder for a while, then slowly experienced my soul slipping back down into my body, a gradual awareness of my chest, torso, and legs, and then, simultaneously, a unified body and soul. I did not open my eyes immediately but basked in an afterglow of tranquility.

Empirical studies conclude that meditation, yoga, and tai chi decrease depression, improve focus and concentration, and help one to cope with stress, all challenges for those with ADHD. ADHD people tend to be highly creative, but often creativity is pushed aside when depression prevails. Creative outlets, such as painting, writing, and music need to be discovered and nurtured, and creativity is often stimulated when one has inner tranquility, which can be accomplished through meditation. In today's fast-paced, highly technological society, we are bombarded with extraneous stimuli: the roar of automobiles, machinery, and our own incessant chatter. If one is perpetually in an active state and running in infinite circles, burnout results, which equals little or no accomplishment.

How often do we take even so much as five minutes from our day to listen to the sounds of silence? Listen to the gurgling of a brook, the water swirling around rocks, the wind rustling through the leaves, the calling of a crow?

Silence in our lives is denied by entertainment, convenience, and comfort.[2] Perls noted that "head chatter" blocks wholeness; silence allows our senses to open, to develop sharper perceptions, and to sharpen acuity.[3] If we are constantly thinking or talking, we miss the richness of the natural world. During a walking meditation class, we wandered in silence on a farm, taking excruciatingly slow steps for forty-five minutes (a feat for me). Not only did time pass quickly, but my visual and auditory senses were heightened. The deep, rich, fertile brown soil in the fields appeared even richer to my eyes. I inhaled the lingering odor of freshly cut grass and listened to the wind whistle through the willow trees. A state of peace enveloped me for hours afterward.

Sometimes a calling or a new direction in life may be heard as a result of silence. When my friend Sherry came with me to meditation one night, she announced that she had decided to move from a town boarding house to a cottage for rent on a friend's horse farm. During meditation, she said the idea suddenly occurred to her. Apparently, she needed that time for reflection to listen to her intuition. I recall my journey to the West Coast and spending long days alone, just being. It was then that art found its way back into my life.

Being can also be a form of meditation, and there are different ways to "be." One method is sitting meditation alone while visualizing an image or chanting a mantra. One can be hiking, observing signs of wildlife or the surrounding vegetation. One can be creating a work of art. It is living within the moment and fully experiencing one's emotions. Clarity of thought and an improved ability to think also come to those engaged in a repetitive, low concentration, physical task such as swimming laps, jogging, or walking.[4] *Being* does not have to imply doing nothing but perhaps involves engagement in an activity conducive to mindfulness.

Meditation teaches mindfulness, one of the directives from Buddhism's Eightfold Path. It is an awareness of the present moment. It demands practice to be utterly present in one's immediate, everyday experience. Meditation can enhance mindfulness, although mindfulness can become an inherent trait practiced during daily tasks. I believe it can also facilitate the Christian doctrine of giving your worries to God, as mindfulness prevents one's thoughts from wandering, thus diminishing worries about the future. If one can live in the present, then one can fully enjoy life. If one lives in the future with worry, then one will not live. Mindfulness can be practiced through any activity, such as gardening, cleaning, or simply washing dishes. For instance, if one is gardening, do not be thinking of what your next task will be or where you need to be later in the day. Concentrate on weeding or planting, crumble the soil between your fingers, carefully examine the intricate webbed pattern of a leaf, feel the breeze tousle your hair, and watch the cloud formations as the sun sets behind the distant pines.

An interesting study revealed that mindfulness is not typically associated with organized religion, but often with back-to-the-landers maintaining small farmsteads who feel a close kinship with nature. Almost half of the study respondents did not claim a religious affiliation (26.6 percent were mainstream Protestants, 17.3 percent conservative Christians, and 12.1 percent Catholics), less than 1 percent were committed to an Eastern or New Age religion, and 81.1 percent indicated that they had a sense of peace of mind. The authors suggested that country life is conducive to mindfulness.[5] However, most of the respondents did not have any prior experience with rural life, so perhaps this suggests a proclivity toward mindfulness to begin with, or an inherent trait that one already possesses. In addition, rural life is quite isolating. Climate conditions, such as snowstorms, often preclude travel throughout the winter. One is likely to attend church on a less frequent basis and to find more informal ways to practice one's beliefs, often through nature or informal get-togethers with friends in the evenings—anything that satiates a spiritual hunger. The study also revealed that these homesteaders were often married or in long-term relationships and had relatively high educational levels.

A life crisis, such as the sudden hospitalization of a loved one or illness, can teach one mindfulness. When my brother was hospitalized for two weeks for surgical removal of a brain tumor, my senses were attuned to every minute. I vividly recall walking down the hallways, aware of every echoing footstep over the diamond-shaped patterns on the brown and pink linoleum tiles. Sometimes when the intensity of my emotions overcame me, I walked to a botanical garden with a small pond and watched the ducklings waddle after their mothers and paddle feverishly through the water, their tiny webbed feet cycling rapidly to keep pace. This tiny oasis on campus was a salvation. At night, in my brother's room in the ICU, I'd drift off to sleep curled up on the window seat, the call bells at the nurse's station echoing in my head. During those arduous and painful days, I did not think beyond the present moment. Every distraction in my life ceased. Mindfulness also teaches the significance of each moment, a greater appreciation of life, and an awareness not to take things for granted. It teaches stillness, creating a vivid awareness of the world around us, heightening our senses. I recall sitting in the courtyard one afternoon, reading a book. Suddenly, I looked up and a great breeze rustled through the trees, turning the leaves to their undersides. God's presence vividly swept through the trees, a gentle hand reminding me of His strength.

Reflecting on death often also teaches mindfulness. No one knows how long we have on this earth. With this awareness in mind, we are driven to savor each day and spend time cultivating and appreciating relationships. This is practicing mindfulness, as well.

Those who practice Theravada meditation refer to ADHD as "monkey mind," or a fickleness in our everyday attention.[6] Only when we recognize this can we begin to practice mindfulness. The goal of samatha, a Buddhist practice, is to still one's mind, which leads to the eventual cessation of thinking and a full awareness of the present.

I first became interested in Buddhism during graduate school when I wrote a paper for my Death and Dying class on Tibetan Buddhist meditation and attended Zen Buddhist lectures conducted by visiting monks. Siddhartha Gautama, known as the Buddha (c. 563-

483 B.C.) founded Buddhism, an international religion, and one without cultural or ethnic bias.[7] In A.D. 527, Bodhidharma traveled from India to China to introduce Buddhism. During the T'ang dynasty (618-907), the Buddhist schools of Pure Land, T'ien-t'ai, Hua-yen, Chen-yen, and Ch'an (Zen) evolved, cultivated by eminent leaders of the time. In the thirteenth century, Buddhist thought was established as Zen in Japan and was depicted in paintings, poetry, calligraphy, swordsmanship, and tea ceremonies. Daisetz Teitaro Suzuki (1870-1966), a professor of Buddhist philosophy at Otani University in Kyoto, brought Zen Buddhism to the West. There are no fixed curricula or standard textbooks to teach a history of classical Zen. During the ninth and tenth centuries in China, the Five Houses arose to teach Zen, represented by several groups of prominent Zen teachers. The Five Houses were not considered sects or schools, and the teachings were not dogmatized. One must personally experience Zen through enlightenment in order to teach it to others. In Zen, concentration and wisdom are the roots of enlightenment. For new learners, they are stopping and seeing.[8] In particular, Buddhism focuses on achieving enlightenment rather than accepting certain dogmas of a faith. I had wanted to explore other religions and formulate my own beliefs rather than commit to a prescribed set of values. Why do we have to subscribe to one set of beliefs? In Buddhism, approaches and methods are adjusted to the needs and capacities of communities and individuals. If one is secure in one's religion, why not adopt and incorporate other practices that are beneficial and will enhance one's spirituality? Cultural pluralism is not practiced or applied enough. Many religious organizations expend too much time and energy condemning other religions for their values, instead of respecting them. If religious organizations focused on the positive qualities that other organizations offered, perhaps barriers would disintegrate and an exchange of ideas would foster growth, instead of stagnation and ill-will toward one another and outside groups. Suzuki stated, "If we feel dissatisfied somehow with this life, if there is something in our ordinary way of living that deprives us of freedom in its most sanctified sense, we must endeavor to find a way somewhere which gives us a sense of finality and contentment."[9]

Japanese Zen students refer to this new perception, or enlightenment, as "satori." Satori may be distinguished from another Buddhist concept known as nirvana. Nirvana is realized when cravings end, when one observes ordinary life as suffering, ensuing from a ceaseless running around in an attempt to satisfy every desire or need. This is typical of those with ADD/ADHD, but it is also quite characteristic of our society and technology. One can achieve liberation only by abandoning these pursuits through escaping such a materialistic life. In contrast, satori does not seek to escape from such a life but, rather, pursues what everyone else does, albeit in another way. In this regard, satori prevents total absorption or entanglement in life that will culminate in suffering. Nirvana and satori both seek to prevent suffering, although each uses different approaches and philosophies.[10]

Satori also arises from two types of consciousness, or knowledge. Vijnana is ordinary knowledge, knowledge of the concrete as well as abstract principles. Prajna is transcendental knowledge that evolves only by cultivating knowledge that leads to satori. It is not abandonment of the ordinary use of the senses or intellect, but looking beyond the limits of the senses. It is undifferentiated and does not focus on any particular goals or objects. Prajna underlies all vijnana, but vijnana is not conscious of prajna; it is sufficient on its own. This is similar to the concept of Freud's philosophy of the id, ego, and superego. The id acts only to satisfy its impulses and does not have any consciousness of the superego that wants to modify the id's behavior. The Zen master concentrates all efforts in awakening prajna that will eventually lead to liberation. In Zen, if prajna is not achieved, then one will never be spiritually fulfilled. If one expends all one's energy on negative thoughts, one can never hope to achieve this liberation.

If one can learn to adopt a different perception of life and thought, perhaps through meditation, art, writing, or music using a Zen-based philosophy, this will be one antidote for depression, especially for those with ADD/ADHD. Adopting a different view of life will help one to break free from the downward spiral of negative thoughts (such as those I depicted in my painting I described in a previous chapter). Furthermore, Buddhism can enhance psychoanalysis.[11,12] Buddhist concepts have taught me much about developing patience and living in the present moment. One of the greatest challenges in Christianity is to learn to relinquish one's worries to God. Worries manifest as anxieties that in turn manifest as illness. Buddhism offers assistance with this task if one learns to focus on the present. If one is focused on the present moment, worries about the future and regrets of the past are soon forgotten. However, it is not the objective of

Zen to be freed from doubts and worries but, rather, to experience these emotions within the self. This is counter to Western philosophy; doctors prescribe Prozac for any bout of depression or loneliness, often the result of an inevitable life event such as death. We are encouraged to run from experiencing our emotions, to hide from pain, but this is the nature of a human being, *Being*. In his article "Repudiation of the Medical Model," Thomas Szasz argues that mental illness does not exist and that psychiatry has failed to accept the fact that human relations are inherently fraught with difficulties.[13] Mental illness is used as an explanation for problems in living and, thus, as an excuse to medicate. In essence, it seems the medical profession believes one should not experience the grief and subsequent depression associated with a loved one's death.

Meditation and mindfulness also teach one to be attentive. Attention is assumed to be automatic and is taken for granted, but it is a learned skill. Samatha, a Buddhist practice, teaches one to develop attention through meditation by focusing on an image, one's breath, objects of meditation, such as a candle, or koans. Koans are logically insoluble riddles, such as "What is the sound of one hand clapping?" The goal of samatha is the eventual cessation of thinking and an awareness of the present moment. This can also be accomplished through physical exercise. When I first started mountain biking, I quickly discovered that I needed to pay close attention to the gnarly roots and logs that quickly appeared in my path. It requires great concentration and skill to maneuver around these obstacles. Because one focuses so intently, all distracting thoughts vanish from the mind. Laura Sewall proposed the concepts of exogenous and endogenous attention.[14] Exogenous attention refers to observation of any immediate changes in our visual field or landscape that may be a potential threat. Endogenous attention refers to a focus on the familiar or what we are primed to see. Evidence suggests that attentional patterns may physically alter the neural pathways in the brain. Structural changes may occur in the visual cortex and strengthen the synaptic connections between neurons, forming new neural associations and pathways. Wilderness experiences are an opportunity to observe with attentiveness what emerges around each bend of the trail, to anticipate what is over each hill.[15]

Eastern tradition focuses on achieving a state of balance and equilibrium between the mind, body, and spirit. Eastern medical philosophy is derived from the observation of living human beings and the relationship between specific symptoms and the body.[16] Western medical study has historically examined specific organs within cadavers, as opposed to observing living human beings. Eastern scientific tradition also focuses on intuition, whereas Western science emphasizes rational thought and the scientific method. Yoga, tai chi, and qigong are examples of such holistic practices. I practiced tai chi for a semester during graduate school and found that after a day of frustration, my spirits immediately lifted. During the class, I focused solely on the movements, which cleared my mind of all distracting thoughts. I often walked back to my apartment enveloped in a great state of tranquility. Intrigued, I started to attend meditation classes and, later, yoga.

Yoga dates back nearly 2,000 years and was first described by Pantajali in the second century in the *Yoga Sutras*. Yoga uses a combination of physical postures and attempts to create an awareness of breath, the self, and energy through meditation. Yoga is derived from the Sanskrit root *yuj* meaning "union" or "yoke."[17] This union is brought about by persistent practice *(abhyasa)* through posture *(asana)*, control of breath *(pranayama)*, concentration *(dharana)*, and meditation *(dhyana)*.

The concept of liberation is central to yoga thought, which may be accomplished when one learns to still the restlessness of the mind. The Sanskrit word *moksa* is often translated into English as freedom or liberation. However, ignorance is believed to be the source of our bondage in the philosophy of yoga. Ignorance imprisons us and hence precludes one from achieving liberation. Through practice one can achieve liberation and thus be released from the bondage of ignorance.

In addition to practice, liberation may also be achieved through detachment, or *vairgya*, a lack of desire for objects. In an interesting essay, Jeffrey Gold draws parallels between yoga and the philosophies of Socrates and Plato. Socrates said that the soul could best reflect when it is free of all such distractions as hearing or sight or pain or pleasure of any kind, when the soul is independent of the body. Plato hypothesized that the soul can reason and think clearly when not distracted by the senses, one of the objectives of yoga. Plato believed that the philosopher must practice separating the soul from the body. Plato viewed the soul as a helpless prisoner, and Socrates claimed that the philosophical soul sought release.[18] Hence, through meditation, one can learn to release the soul and, in turn, be freed from ignorance.

Hatha yoga seeks to free people from physical limitations and to restore balance to the body. Different types of hatha yoga include Ashtanga, Iyengar, Integral, and Kripalu. Hatha yoga is said to balance the hemispheres of the brain. "Ha" means sun and "tha" means moon. One hemisphere tends to dominate our actions and thought. Mathematicians and scientists are more likely to employ left-brain thinking, which controls logic and rationale. Artists, writers, and musicians are more likely to use the right side of the brain, which is responsible for creativity. The corpus callosum connects the two hemispheres together, but many of us do not often use this passageway to the other side, which could enhance our work. Practice of hatha yoga may enable us to simultaneously use both hemispheres. Ancient Chinese and Greek traditions promote balance as the key to longevity and health. Balance is restored through a unification of the physical body, breath, and concentration.

The Chinese believe that a balance between yin and yang will restore health. This balances energy in the body known as qi, or ch'i. Yin and yang are the two opposing forces present in all of creation, including in people and herbs. Yang represents warmth, brightness, dominance, and masculinity. Yin represents coolness, dimness, yielding, and femininity. According to Chinese Taoism, excessive stress and anxiety can result in a yin deficiency. The Taoist religion originated from the Chinese observations of balance and opposites working together in harmony, a native spiritual tradition that emulated Buddhism. Stress and anxiety are comorbid symptoms of ADHD. Perhaps those with ADHD tend to exhibit an excess of yang characteristics, as well as deficiencies in yin characteristics.

Balance is also found in nature. The Chinese viewed the movement from night to day and winter to summer as forming a rhythmic union. Rhythmic unions are found everywhere in nature. Farming has taught me to live and work within the seasons, and this has created a balance for me. One learns to plant certain fruits and vegetables during the spring, summer, and fall and thus consume what is in season. One becomes excited when picking blueberries in the summer, harvesting butternut squash in the fall, and planting tomatoes and peppers in late spring. One learns to go to bed with the moon and rise with the sun, following the philosophy of hatha yoga. Drawing and painting as a form of meditation also teaches balance and simultaneous use of both hemispheres of the brain. It is commonly thought that artists typically use the right brain hemisphere because the left hemisphere involves rational thinking, which can hinder the creative process. *Drawing on the Artist Within* by Betty Edwards teaches exercises to balance and simultaneously employ both hemispheres.[19]

Hatha yoga focuses on breathing techniques *(pranayama)* and movement. Physical postures *(asanas)* are performed while standing, sitting, or lying on the floor. Each joint in the body moves through a full range of strengthening, balancing, and stretching. Focusing on the bodily sensations through the acts of exhaling and inhaling improves attention and will help one to focus on tasks in daily life, pay attention to body cues, maintain a sense of relaxation, and slow down thoughts. Breathing techniques focus on prolonged inhalation, breath retention, and exhalation. Common yoga techniques include conscious breathing in the lower, middle, and upper portions of the lungs; interval breathing, in which inhalations and exhalation are altered; and alternate nostril breathing. Alternate nostril breathing balances hemispheric asymmetry in electroencephalogram (EEG) waves.[20]

Yoga, as a form of meditation, boosts energy and improves memory and concentration, often problems afflicting those with ADD/ADHD. Yoga also promotes strength, endurance, and flexibility through bodily sensations and decreases negative emotions such as anger, fear, and hate.[21] Yoga students develop coping skills for eating disorders, drug use, and low-grade depression. Physical benefits include relaxing the nervous system and improving memory and concentration. Yoga also improves digestion; stimulates the pancreas, liver, gall bladder, spleen, bladder, and gonads; increases circulation; regulates menstrual irregularities; helps irrigate kidneys; and relaxes the nervous system.[22] Studies also report an association between yoga and reduction in body weight.[23]

Yoga utilizes the parasympathetic nervous system to aid in calming the body. During a crisis, one can apply the skills developed in yoga and meditation. Some studies conclude that meditation relieves stress-related disease; decreases stress-related complaints, such as headaches, gastritis, and insomnia; decreases blood pressure during practice; and enables one to maintain lower blood pressure.[24] As previously mentioned in Chapter 1, Sudarshana Kriya Yoga (SKY), when practiced as a sole treatment for thirty minutes daily for three months, increased P300 wave amplitude (brain waves that are found to be decreased in those with ADD/ADHD) and also improved symptoms of dysthymia, normalizing at three months.[25]

Meditation, through any of the practices discussed in this chapter, is a form of dissociation, a normal and natural cognitive function. Dissociation occurs when we progressively disconnect from the external world and attend to internal images, memories, and impressions.[26] The simple act of focusing or concentrating attention involves a degree of dissociation. Painting and writing are forms of dissociation, and I often use them as meditation practice. It is not any different from focusing on a visual image in my mind, and I do not think of anything else except what is before me on the canvas. I become so absorbed in painting that I am oblivious to the presence of anyone in the room and will often neglect to eat. Although some psychologists refer to this as "hyperfocusing," a symptom of ADD/ADHD, it is meditation or a dissociative state, which I believe comes with ease for many artists, writers, and musicians.

Intuition is a wisdom that may be developed through the introspective practices of yoga, tai chi, or meditation, among others. In turn, this may enhance one's painting, writing, or music. Intuition is recognizing an inner voice and listening to that voice during times of tribulation and indecision. Intuition, along with faith, may help one to find a calling in life.

Chapter 8

Paths to Destinations Unknown

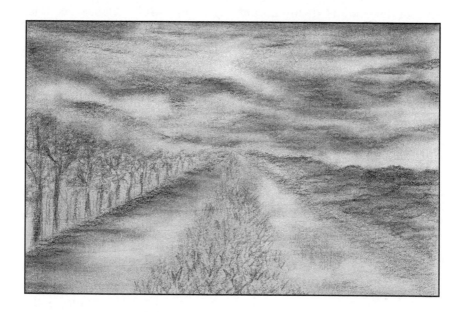

If one advances confidently in the direction of his dreams and endeavors to live the life which he has imagined, he will meet with a success unexpected in common hours. . . . If you have built castles in the air, your work need not be lost; that is where they should be. Now put the foundations under them.

Henry David Thoreau

It is midway through the summer and I am sitting under a canopy of foliage, green apples clinging to branchlets. A fleeting memory of fall comes to mind, when I collected fallen apples and brought them to school. We cranked apples through an old press, students ecstatically taking turns to grind the apples into cider. On this farm where I live, the orchard is bursting with new growth. Apples, peaches, pears, and plums dangle from nearby trees, still in the early stages of growth. The cherry tree boasts tart fruit ripe for picking and baking cobbler. Thorny blackberry bushes do not prevent me from plucking as many berries as I can.

Daylilies surround blooming cosmos; strawflowers and four o'clocks mix in the borders of my garden. The first sunflower has debuted, stretching its bright yellow petals, and a bee nuzzles into the brown disk. A rectangular border of sunflowers frames the herb gardens and strawberry patch. The tomato plants are beginning to bear succulent Sungold cherry tomatoes, and the Brandywines are slowly appearing, green, but soon to evolve into plump, pink fruit. A salsa pepper dangles from a nearby pepper plant. Green sheaves of cornstalks wave in the breeze, and it is exciting to watch the evolution of surrounding cornfields from my bicycle. Green stalks of Evergreen onion and Mars red onion shoot upward, and luminescent yellow flowers blossom on zucchini and patty pan squash plants. Here and there, burdock and thistle poke their heads through layers of hay mulch donated from the barn of my landlords to smother weeds and retain moisture in the soil. Walt has kindly offered me space at his roadside stand to sell my vegetables.

Immersing myself in nature has inspired many of my paintings and writings. Wandering through forests often leads to inquisitive questions about trees, vegetation, and wildlife. Studying the texture of the bark of an apple tree inspires a painting, which in turn invokes the study of color theory, mixing innumerable varieties of grays, browns, and greens.

Creativity *is* a gift, but one that needs to be nurtured or it ultimately falls into addiction. During the storms of life, it is inherently therapeutic to sit down to write, paint, or play music. It is a journey as well, one that can be traversed many ways, but it can be a long, lonely journey at times; this solitude is necessary for creation. A painting of mine, titled *paths to destinations unknown,* portrays a bicycle towpath next to a canal. One unusually warm December afternoon, I biked along a canal. Lilac and fiery amber clouds streaked the sky and the towpath and canal converged together in the distance. There are many ways to travel to this converging point, this destination in our lives, whatever it may be. One can choose the graveled towpath or the cool canal waters.

There are choices that lie within each as well. One may bike, walk, or run along the towpath, canoe, kayak, or swim the canal. Each path chosen will be an inherently unique experience, although all paths ultimately reach the same destination. It is the journey and the way we choose to travel it that matter. If you pedal as fast as you can, you are guaranteed to miss hidden treasures along the way. Walking, or doing one of these other activities in a slower manner, enables you to discover those hidden riches, and this also includes relationships. Relationships and nature, together, contribute to creativity, enhancing and shaping it. This book would not exist were it not for my family and friends who contributed to it.

When I first plunged into painting and writing, I focused solely on the destination, eventually working only for productivity. Inevitably, I stopped enjoying it, as well as the relationships with people in my life. Farming and hiking taught me to savor every day, to relish the joys found along a trail or in the fields. In my garden the other day, I discovered random plum tomatoes that had sprouted from last year's seeds, concealed under the sunflowers, a variety called Evening Sun that boasted wine-stained and crimson-colored petals. The plum tomatoes were a gift, as I could not care for my plum tomato seedlings during my brother's illness. Often, a painting or some writing evolves from these discoveries, and I simply enjoy it, forgetting about where I will sell it or what show to enter. I would rather give it as a gift to family or friends or sell it to those who understand the underlying emotions.

Once upon a time, I shoved innumerable drawings under my bed and journals of poetry in a drawer—perhaps afraid they would be shunned by others or in fear of revealing true emotions. Only in the past few years have I begun to share these with friends and family, and it brings great fulfillment to elicit emotion and memorable experiences. This truly is the gift of creativity. Creativity is also an educational tool. Activism assumes many forms, and one can use art, music, or writing to advocate for one's convictions, whether they are for environmental concerns or social issues. Artists can educate others through paintings about organic farming, poets can write about the earth, and musicians can sing about homelessness. This is only a small sample of the infinite ways to use one's creativity. Creativity may be found in a calling or a calling may be found from creativity. Perhaps your calling is to teach your creativity, whether it be art, music, or writing, but you are nurturing creativity in yourself, as well as others. Sparking creativity and nurturing it in another is the greatest gift one can give back to others.

I recently returned from a writer's conference at Calvin College in Grand Rapids, Michigan, held every two years. My mother's friend, Anne, had encouraged me to travel 740 miles with my mother for three days of seminars. I had no expectations prior to leaving, but my restlessness prompted a needed excursion.

After a long and arduous drive, Anne welcomed us with warm hospitality and served a wonderful Thai dinner and wine. Satiated, we slept well and drove to the college early the next morning. The campus swarmed with hundreds of people and the morning began with an array of seminars. Professors from prominent colleges and universities around the country convened to contrast beloved authors such as C. S. Lewis, J. R. R. Tolkien, Thoreau, and Emerson. A playwright from New York staged her play, *As It Is in Heaven,* about a Shaker community that is torn apart when a newcomer suddenly sees visions of angels and views herself as an instrument of God. Another member of the community began to draw trees from visions in her head, claiming her art to be a gift from God, and she, a mere instrument. Michael Card, a contemporary Christian musician, spoke at a workshop and further elaborated on this concept. Artists produce artifacts, the *tangible* outcomes of our creativity, but we are not our gifts. Our creativity far surpasses our comprehension.

At the end of the conference, I picked up a copy of Madeleine L'Engle's book, *Walking on Water: Reflections on Faith and Art.* L'Engle draws the analogy of a "lake of creativity" and every artist must contribute to this lake whether it is a river or a trickle. Each drop counts. I am only one person and I could continue to push paintings under my bed, but I would not be making any contributions to the world. And if everyone felt this way, the lake would dry up. What would today be like without art, music, poetry, or literature? As artists, we record history, tell stories, express emotions, and advocate our convictions with our gifts of creativity. For so many years, I cursed my creativity and felt it selfish to focus solely on writing and painting. What I realized during the conference is that it was selfish of me *not* to pursue my gifts of creativity.

However, for many years, I found it very difficult to thoroughly enjoy someone's response to my paintings or writing. What did they know about it, I'd ponder angrily. But inevitably, it dawned on me that it did not matter. What mattered is that they derived joy, inspiration, or thought from it. And that was my gift to them. Slowly, I started to truly enjoy someone's response to my art, but this only occurred when I began to accept and appreciate myself. Appreciating someone's response to my work only happened when I allowed others to love me.

paths to destinations unknown, as well as this book, is also about finding a calling in life. A calling is complex to define, but it is your sense of purpose in life, your place, your direction, perhaps discovered through listening to God, to your intuition, or through a meditative experience. Maybe it is somewhat of a preconceived destiny based on your creative gifts, if you stumble upon it after asking for it through prayer or meditation. However, some hear a calling very early in life, and there is little doubt as to their life direction. Still others experience a sudden illness that changes their life direction, often for the better. It may take years before one finds a calling, perhaps after venturing down many a path and having many life experiences, but it is often these experiences that prepare us for a calling heard later in life. There may be those who profess not to have heard a calling, but perhaps they choose not to listen.

Often those diagnosed with ADD/ADHD may struggle the most to hear a calling or find a calling because of a restless nature that prevents them from listening. If one is blessed with many creative gifts, it is often difficult to determine a life direction and what type of career is best suited for a restless, energetic, and creative personality. It is also difficult to find focus before and even after one finds a calling in life, as distractibility will remain an eternal problem. Even when one finds a calling, one can still be scattered and, as a result, not be very successful because one's attention is too divided.

My brother has recently started his own nondenominational church, and for a while, was renting a converted barn on Fellowship Farm in Pottstown, Pennsylvania. My family and I attended the outdoor Easter morning service, a gathering of over eighty people under an outdoor pavilion. After the service, I wandered over with my little cousins, Anna and Nicky, to watch a goat nuzzling some grass by a wire fence. The goat continued to nibble, his nose slowly poking through the bottom of the fence. Suddenly, he extended his neck and started to crawl out, but the fence prevented him from going farther. He appeared trapped, but contentedly continued to munch on the grass outside the fence. For a minute, we worried that he was ensnared by the fence, but my mother pointed out how worn this particular grass plot was.

"Obviously he's done this before," she commented.

"Why? Look at this entire yard he has to graze on!" I said.

Even before the words escaped my mouth, I realized the impact of what I had just said. I had attended some of the Bible study sessions Chris had organized and we had read a book by Philip Keller, *A Shepherd Looks at Psalm 23*. Although this book focused on a shepherd's experience tending sheep, the same analogy could be applied to this particular goat.

Keller writes, "In spite of having such a master and owner, the fact remains that some Christians are still not content with His control. They are somewhat dissatisfied, always feeling that somehow the grass beyond the fence must be a little greener. These are carnal Christians— one might almost call them "fence crawlers" or "half Christians" who want the best of both worlds."[1]

He continues to discuss one particular sheep. "She was simply never contented with things as they were. Often when she had forced her way through some such spot in a fence or found a way around the end of the wire at low tide on the beaches, she would end up feeding on bare, brown, burned-up pasturage of a most inferior sort. But she never learned her lesson and continued to fence crawl time after time."[2]

Although I do believe some restlessness may be attributed to physiological explanations, perhaps there is some truth to Keller's analogy. There may be particular paths in life that we are destined to follow and when we deviate from them, there are ramifications. I have observed these patterns in my life. When I leave a particular job or school that I feel I am meant to be at, my life quickly deteriorates. Things do not work out. Sometimes I have had the chance to return and rectify my abrupt departure and things suddenly resolve themselves. Perhaps this involves learning to stay focused and not be attracted by the innumerable distractions in life.

Focus can be established through meditation, solitude, and organization. With focus comes ambition. One who suddenly seemed to lack any ambition may suddenly become ambitious once they discover a calling.

Others with ADD/ADHD may struggle to find a calling because they resent authority and do not want to be taught anything. I majored in art in college for *one* day because I did not want to be told what to draw or how to do it. Of course, years later I would kick myself for being foolishly ignorant, and I know that my art may have greatly evolved over the past ten years had I been open to being taught. However, it was something that I needed to learn on my own, and I find that many diagnosed with ADD/ADHD are self-taught, successful artists, writers, and musicians for the very same reason. But it takes persistence, dedication, and self-discipline. If you so desire something and stand by your convictions, then, by all means, do not lose sight of your dreams. My philosophy has been to cast my line out often and anywhere to see what bites. Simply talking to others at a social gathering or joining organizations as a volunteer may lead to a job and eventually a calling that may alleviate depression and addiction problems. One solution is to find autonomy within a career, one that does not shackle you to a desk. News reporting allows one to investigate social and news events, and teaching grants creative freedom. Or initiate a business that allows you to use your hands, whether it is starting a CSA, landscaping, construction, catering, or home improvements. Autonomy grants the opportunity to achieve one's potential because it entails a sense of freedom and of liberation. One takes pride in building something of one's own, whether it is in the literal or figurative sense.

Callings do imply commitment, a trait with which many creative people struggle. Restlessness and commitment are of a dichotomous nature, and one is confronted with the dilemma of pursuing a calling and abandoning a restless nature. But as I stated earlier, rootedness does not imply immobility. We can still retain freedom, although we are never truly free from any responsibility, regardless of the path we pursue. It is wise to stay committed to a calling as other paths you may so choose will have obstacles. God granted us free will, but He also prepares those who seek or hear a calling. This calling may be teaching, caring for a loved one, or preaching and ministering to others. When one decides to follow a calling, the details simply fall into place. As Stewart once said, "God will provide." It is natural to experience resentment when a sense of commitment or obligation restricts freedom, but the benefits derived from a calling far surpass the disadvantages. In a sense, a calling restores freedom. It may allow you to pursue other passions in life and have the security of a job, or it may grant opportunities to explore other areas of study.

Having an obstinate personality will be of great assistance because often this evolves into persistence. Persistence, as well as faith, leads to accomplishment. Assume risk in life. Start an organization. Seek out alternative, progressive schools where people will appreciate your creative gifts and energy, rather than emphasize flaws or stress strictures such as organization or time management. I have even found those who appreciate these quirky traits. Teach others who suffer from depression once you have conquered yours. Guide them and watch them blossom. People who have made the greatest impact in my life were teachers or those who took only a few hours out of their day to talk and listen. Even volunteering to teach a workshop for a week or working on a mission trip can touch someone else for a lifetime, although we may never realize the impact that we have. Growing up, my father introduced us to artists and taught my brother and I how to draw on weekends while sitting at the dining room table with us, sketching portraits and sailboats, one of his passions. At bedtime, he wove elaborate, impromptu tales. Before pursuing a career in the ministry, my brother worked as an architect, and I have become an oil painter, thanks to the support of my parents, who provided me with paints, brushes, and books. After many detours in his career life, my father has been teaching history and art in public and private high schools for the past seven years, and his face lights up when he speaks of a student or a new project. I am very grateful to my mother who persistently dragged us to church and on mission trips to build houses, and who provided a strong sense of community. We often joke with our parents that we were raised in a bed-and-breakfast, one with a revolving door open to guest after guest.

I am eternally grateful to Kim Pearson, my undergraduate advisor and writing professor, for the foundation she built for me. Initially, I majored in English, but conflicts with English professors prompted me to only minor in Professional Writing. Kim Pearson taught me to write. She demanded revision after revision. Often, it discouraged me and I thought I fell short of her expectations. But she challenged me as no one else ever had before. And once I abandoned my insecurities and resistance, my writing improved.

A dynamic, petite African-American woman in long braids, Kim energetically paced the room, talking excitedly about the latest speaker she was bringing in, or the magazine article or business plan she had assigned for us to write. She had great vision, despite battling health problems and personal obstacles. She grew up poverty-stricken amid the race riots in Philadelphia during the 1960s and vowed to change the world through teaching. During my junior year, Kim's health deteriorated, and she became confined to a wheelchair. She suffered from ankylosing spondylitis, a rare spinal disease that permanently stiffened her backbone. In spite of this affliction, she continued to teach and mentored two of my independent studies, teaching me to write and expand my research. Recently, I learned that she was named New Jersey Professor of the Year, no doubt as to why. I contacted her and she invited me to sit in on her current Introduction to Professional Writing course, just as I had ten years ago as a sophomore. With the help of recent surgery, she was once again walking energetically across the room, her face breaking into its characteristic grin, her eyes sparkling when she caught hold of an idea.

She now incorporated an element of activism, eliciting a philosophical discussion on a current campus issue that had sparked much debate. She assigned students to write letters to a particular corporation that monetarily supported sweatshops, thus teaching her students to find an active voice in society and a way to creatively express themselves. We are not merely observers or passive recipients of events that impact our lives. Perhaps this will spark a desire in some of her students to pursue careers in politics, news reporting, writing, activism, or social work. It is a pedagogical approach that provokes thought, stimulates creativity, creates awareness of prevalent social issues, and teaches students to generate pragmatic solutions that will make a difference. This is the concept of ecological literacy. Kim also has created and manages an online news magazine that is run by students and the community. She is also working to initiate a nonprofit academic summer program for inner-city high school students who will have the opportunity to learn and practice journalism through reporting, writing, editing, and producing a magazine issue, and to work with after-school programs in their home communities and eventually with professional media and e-commerce firms. Above all else, Kim Pearson teaches persistence and dedication. Calvin Coolidge said, "The world is full of educated derelicts. Persistence and determination alone are omnipotent. Press on!"

Finally, it is faith that will help you accomplish your goals and weather the storms in life. During some recent turbulent times, my brother handed me the Bible, opened to the Book of Job.

I must have looked at him with a weary expression, because he said, affirmatively, "Just read it."

And so I did.

"One day when Job's children were having a feast at the home of their oldest brother, a messenger came running to Job. 'We were plowing the fields with the oxen,' he said, 'and the donkeys were in a nearby pasture. Suddenly the Sabeans [supernatural beings who serve God in heaven] attacked and stole them all. They killed every one of your servants except me. I am the only one who escaped to tell you'" (Job 1:13-15). The parable continues until all of Job's children and wealth are destroyed. "Then Job got up and tore his clothes in grief. He shaved his head and threw himself face downward on the ground. He said, 'I was born with nothing, and I will die with nothing. The Lord gave, and now he has taken away. May his name be praised!' In spite of everything that had happened, Job did not sin by blaming God" (Job 1:20-22). Furthermore, Job says to his wife when she chastises him for remaining faithful to God, "'When God sends us something good, welcome it. How can we complain when he sends us trouble?' Even in all this suffering Job said nothing against God" (Job 2:10). However, Job eventually complains to God and curses the day he was born. God answers his prayers and blesses Job with twice as much as he had before, including seven sons, three daughters, and a multitude of livestock.

Troubles will always afflict us, but faith is a life preserver. Especially for those blessed with creativity. We meet people in life at particular times who offer guidance and hope; these relationships may serve a purpose for a few days, years, or a lifetime. But it is your faith and creative gifts that will encourage you to keep swimming, running, walking, kayaking, hiking, whatever mode of transportation helps you to traverse those paths to destinations unknown.

Appendix A

Environmental Education Resources

Activity Ideas

- Volunteer to work in a community garden. Call city/town hall and find out if there are any community gardens or write a brief proposal to turn a vacant lot into a garden and present it at a town meeting.
- Volunteer or find a paid internship on a farm or nature preserve. Type "environmental education" or "nature preserves/centers" in the search area of an Internet search engine such as Yahoo, Alta Vista, or Web-Crawler.
- Start a community garden/composting program in your school on any size land using gardening resources listed in Appendix B or ask a friend/educator knowledgeable in gardening to help out. Basic tools required are shovels, rakes, hand trowels, and seed packets or seed-lings (can be purchased from nurseries or farms). Garden centers also donate leftovers at the end of the year.
- Contact university cooperative extensions (established by the U.S. Department of Agriculture based on the Smith-Lever Act of 1914) for gardening and composting resources (e.g., Penn State and Rutgers University).
- Organize field trips to local nature centers and farms. Some farms offer one- to two-hour programs that teach youths farming basics. Nature centers offer year-round programs and workshops for educators and students at nominal costs. Programs may include stream/forest ecology, entomology, wildlife, birds, and sugar maple tapping.

Environmental Organizations

Join/volunteer or start an environmental organization. Suggestions:

- **The Green Party:** First established in 1973 in most European countries. Dedicated to promoting ecological wisdom, social justice, non-violence, decentralization, sustainability, and feminism through a grassroots democracy. Web site: <http://www.greenparty.org>.

- **The Sierra Club:** Founded by John Muir in the nineteenth century to promote land conservation, wildlife, and outdoor adventures. Web site: <http://www.sierraclub.org>.
- **Trees Forever:** Published the Tree Project Handbook, a Volunteer Action Guide for planting trees in the community and organizing volunteers. Phone: 800-369-1269 or 319-373-0650; 1233 7th Avenue, Marion, Iowa 52302.
- **Greenpeace,** 1436 U Street NW, Washington, DC 20009.
- **Worldwatch Institute,** 1776 Massachusetts Avenue NW, Washington, DC 20036.
- **Earth Force Programs:** Created in 1993 by The Pew Charitable Trusts. The Youth Advisory Board (YAB) is comprised of fifteen members, ages twelve to seventeen. The YAB recently finished the successful Get Out Spoke'n campaign that encouraged bike-friendly communities. Two other programs include Community Action and Problem Solving (CAPS) to help middle school students identify local environmental issues and implement sustainable action plans. The Global Rivers Environmental Education Network (GREEN) teaches youths to develop local programs to conserve and protect vital water resources. Contact: Jean Wallace, Director of Education, 215-884-9888; Web site: <http://www.earthforce.org>.
- **National Arbor Day Foundation:** Offers activities for Arbor Day and seed packets with instructions for planting seeds. Web site: <http://www.arborday.org>.

Suggested Ecology Books

Berry, Thomas, *The Dream of the Earth* (San Francisco, CA: The Sierra Club, 1988).
Berry, Wendell, *The Gift of Good Land* (Canada: HarperCollins Canada Ltd., 1981).
Berry, Wendell, *Sex, Economy, Freedom and Community* (New York: Pantheon Books, 1992).
Berry, Wendell, *The Unsettling of America: Culture and Agriculture* (San Francisco, CA: The Sierra Club, 1977).
Carson, Rachel, *Silent Spring* (New York: Fawcett World Library, 1962).
Devall, Bill and Sessions, George, *Deep Ecology* (Layton, UT: Gibbs Smith Publisher, 1986).
Donahue, Brian, *Reclaiming the Commons: Community Farms and Forests in a New England Town* (New Haven, CT: Yale University Press, 1999).
Du Nann Winter, Deborah, *Ecological Psychology* (New York: HarperCollins, 1996).

Ehrenfeld, David, *Beginning Again: People and Nature in the New Millennium* (New York: Oxford University Press, 1995).

Heinrich, Bernd, *The Trees in My Forest* (New York: Cliff Street Books, 1997).

Henderson, Elizabeth with Van En, Robyn, *Sharing the Harvest: A Guide to Community-Supported Agriculture* (White River Junction, VT: Chelsea Green Publishing, 1999).

Jackson, Wes, *Becoming Native to This Place* (Lexington, KY: The University Press of Kentucky, 1994).

Jackson, Wes, *New Roots for Agriculture* (Lincoln, NE: University of Nebraska Press, 1985).

Logsdon, Gene, *The Contrary Farmer* (White River Junction, VT: Chelsea Green Publishing, 1994).

Muir, John, *The Wilderness World of John Muir* (Boston, MA: Mariner Books, 2001).

Nearing, Helen and Scott, *Living the Good Life* (New York: Schocken Books, 1970).

Nearing, Helen and Scott, *The Maple Sugar Book* (New York: Schocken Books, 1970).

Orr, David, *Earth in Mind* (Washington, DC: Island Press, 1994).

Orr, David, *Ecological Literacy: Education and the Transition to a Postmodern World* (Albany, NY: State University of New York Press, 1992).

Perrin, Noel, *The Amateur Sugar Maker* (Hanover, NH: University Press of New England, 1972).

Perrin, Noel, *(First, Second, Third) Person Rural* (New York: Penguin Books, 1985).

Roszak, Theodore, Gomes, Mary, and Kannes, Allan, *Ecopsychology: Restoring the Earth, Healing the Mind* (San Francisco, CA: The Sierra Club, 1995).

Sewall, Laura, *Sight and Sensibility: The Ecopsychology of Perception* (New York: Tarcher/Putnam Books, 1999).

Thomashow, Mitchell, *Ecological Identity: Becoming a Reflective Environmentalist* (Boston, MA: MIT Press, 1996).

Thoreau, Henry David, *Walden* (Ware, Hertfordshire: Wordsworth Editions Ltd, 1995).

Wilson, Edward, *Biophilia* (Boston, MA: Harvard University Press, 1984).

Worster, Donald, *Nature's Economy* (Boston, MA: Cambridge University Press, 1994).

Book Resources for Teaching

Burnie, David, Farndon, John, and Allaby, Michael. *How Nature [the Earth, the Weather] Works: 100 Ways Parents and Kids Can Share the*

Secrets of Nature [the Earth, the Weather]. 1991-1995. Reader's Digest, Pleasantville, NY.

Council for Environmental Education. *Project WILD: Environmental Activities for K-12.* 1992, 1985, 1983. Web site: <http://www.eelink.umich.edu/wild/>.

The Earthworks Group. *50 Simple Things You Can Do to Save the Earth.* 1989. Earthworks Press, Berkeley, CA.

Green Teacher, P.O. Box 1431, Lewiston, NY 14092. A resourceful magazine that focuses on environmental awareness.

PLT Activity Guide, a publication of Project Learning Tree for grades K-6 and 7-12. Write to the American Forest Council, 1250 Connecticut Avenue, NW, Washington, DC 20036. Prepared lessons on the environment, forests, food, and democracy.

Sheehan, Kathryn and Waidner, Mary. *Earth Child: Games, Stories, Activities, Experiments and Ideas About Living Lightly on the Earth.* 1991, 1994. Council Oak Books, Tulsa, OK.

Field Guides

Buy/borrow field guides to learn to identify trees, insects, flowers, pond/stream life. Simply start by walking around your own backyard with one of these pictorial guides:

The Peterson Field Guide Series (Birds, Birds' Nests, Eastern Trees, Wildflowers, Ferns, Mammals, Animal Tracks, Reptiles and Amphibians, Insects, Butterflies, Moths, Beetles, Shells, Edible Wild Plants, Mushrooms, Eastern Forests, Seashore, Coastal Fishes, Coral Reefs, Rocks and Minerals, Atmosphere, Stars and Planets), 1998. Houghton Mifflin, Boston, MA.

Reader's Digest North American Wildlife. Reader's Digest, 1998. Pleasantville, NY.

Walker, Laurence C., *Forests, A Naturalist's Guide to Trees and Forest Ecology.* 1990. John Wiley and Sons, New York.

Environmental Programs and Internships

- **Stony Brook Millstone Watershed Association:** 31 Pennington Road, Pennington, NJ 08534. Phone: 609-737-7592. Web site: <http://www.thewatershed.org>. Contact: Rick Lear, Educational Director. Incredible internship program as a teacher/naturalist that offers two weeks of intensive ecology training, teaching experience, and research opportunities during the fall, spring, or summer sessions.

- **AmeriCorps:** A nine-month internship that includes a stipend for living expenses or loan reimbursements; offers national internships in urban areas to teach environmental education (e.g., community gardening, water conservation) or promote social justice (e.g., help people obtain low-income housing). Web site: <http://americorps.org>.
- **PeaceCorps:** Two-year national/international internships in teaching, social work, and environmental education. Web site: <http://www.peacecorps.gov>.
- **Redcliff Ascent Wilderness Treatment Program:** Web site: <http://www.redcliffascent.com>.
- **4-H:** Local and national chapters offering urban and rural community service projects that provide active learning interaction between youths and adults in communication, leadership, career development, livestock, home improvement, and computer technology. Web site: <http://www.4-H.org/fourhweb/statelist.htm>.
- **Association for Experiential Education:** Online journal, conferences, and workshops. Web site: <http://www.aee.org>.
- **Earth Force:** Program started in 1993 by the Pew Charitable Trusts to help schools and community groups focus on local environmental issues and initiate projects. A national Youth Advisory Board (YAB), comprised of fifteen youths ages twelve to seventeen, helps direct Earth Force. A recent campaign focused on bike-friendly communities. Web site: <http://www.earthforce.org>.
- **Community Action and Problem Solving (CAPS):** Program started by Earth Force that helps middle school students identify an environmental issue in their community through research and implement a sustainable action plan. Earth Force has established sites to initiate CAPS in places across the nation, including Chicago, IL, Charleston, SC, Denver, CO, Erie and Philadelphia, PA, Portland, OR, and West Palm Beach and the Tampa Bay/St. Petersburg area, FL. See the Earth Force Web site listed previously for more information.

Appendix B

Agricultural Resources
for Teaching or Internships

- Contact the **National Gardening Association** for resources and an excellent monthly journal featuring an exchange of gardening ideas from nationwide educators. Annually offers $750 worth of gardening products, tools, and seeds to 400 youth gardens nationwide for educators working with at least fifteen children between the ages of three and eighteen years. Phone: 800-538-7476. Web site: <http://www. garden.org>.
- Contact the **Rodale Institute** for resources and books, if not a visit; 333-acre organic farm in Kutztown, PA, dedicated to teaching youths and educators through public programs on the benefits of organic farming and food. The farm is breathtakingly beautiful and features a large apple orchard, museum, bookstore, herb garden, and community-supported agriculture program. Phone: 610-683-1400. E-mail: info@rodaleinst.org. Web site: <http://www.rodaleinstitute.org>.
- **Northeast Organic Farming Association (NOFA).** Web site: <http://www.nofa.org/index.html>.
- **American Horticultural Society**. Web site: <http://www.ahs.org>.
- **The Food Project**. Web site: <http://www.thefoodproject.org>.
- **America the Beautiful Fund:** Offers between 100 and 1,000 seed packets on the basis of need. Call 1-800-522-3557 to request an application.
- **Community Development Block Grants:** Federal funds of $500 to $50,000 distributed to cities to develop gardens. Contact your local mayor's office.
- **PA Department of Education, Office of Environment and Ecology:** Offers grants up to $5,000 per school for gardening, recycling, and composting programs. Contact your state department of education to see what they offer. The PA Department of Education also provides complimentary Earth Day programs and a comprehensive forest ecology activity kit called Sustaining Penn's Woods that includes videos and a variety of experiential activities selected from national cur-

riculum projects for middle and high school students. Phone: 717-783-6994. Web site: <http://www.pde.psu.edu>.

- **USDA Sustainable Agriculture Research and Education (SARE):** Program works to increase knowledge and help farmers adopt practices that are economically viable and that enhance quality of life for farmers, rural communities, and society as a whole. Began funding competitive grants in 1988. Since then, it has funded more than 1,200 projects aimed at improving the sustainability of farming. Phone: 802-656-0471.
- **Biodynamic Farming and Gardening Association:** Call 800-516-7797 to request a list of community-supported agriculture (CSA) programs for your state. Web site: <http://www.biodynamic.com>.
- **University of Guelph, Ontario, Canada:** Offers the Ontario Diploma in Agriculture, many other certificates, and credit and noncredit classes in independent study in agriculture and horticulture. Room 010, Johnston Hall, Guelph, Ontario, N1G 2W1. Phone: 519-767-5050. Web site: <http://www.uoguelph.ca/istudy>.
- **Pennsylvania Association of Sustainable Agriculture (PASA):** Highly resourceful and dynamic organization; organizes an annual two-day conference of seminars and workshops for farmers and educators. P.O. Box 419, 114 West Main Street, Millheim, PA 16854. Web site: <http://www.pasa.org>.
- **Plant A Row (PAR) Program:** Feed the hungry and plant a row in your garden to donate to a local food bank. Phone: 877-492-2727. Web site: <http://www.gwaa.org>.
- **The Land Institute:** Founded by Wes Jackson, a plant geneticist who developed natural systems agriculture, or perennial polyculture, focuses on replacing today's annual crops—corn, wheat, and soybeans—with perennials that will hopefully restore some of the ecological functions of the vanished grasslands of the Midwestern United States. The Land Institute has also established Sunshine Farm, a ten-year project devoted to growing livestock and conventional crops without fossil fuels, chemicals, or irrigation, as well as the Rural Community Studies Center to incorporate ecology into the curricula of local schools. The institute also issues grants to graduate students. 2440 E. Water Well Road, Salina, KS 67401. Phone: 785-823-5376. Web site: <http://www.LandInstitute.org>.
- **Center for Ecoliteracy:** California's Department of Education dedicated to "a garden in every school." Call 916-323-2473 to request a complimentary guide with step-by-step instructions on starting a school garden project. Nutrition Services Division, 560 J Street, Room 270, Sacramento, CA 95814.

- **Agriculture in the Classroom:** Publishes *The Resource Guide to Educational Material About Agriculture.* Order a complimentary copy by contacting STOP 2291, Room 3920-S, 1400 Independence Avenue, SW, Washington, DC 20250-0991.
- **Center for Sustainable Agriculture, UVM:** Publishes *From A to Z in Sustainable Agriculture: A Curriculum Directory for Grades K-12.* 1995. University of Vermont, Burlington, VT. Provides resources and contacts for educational materials on sustainable agriculture. Contact Elizabeth Seyler, Coordinator, 590 Main Street, Burlington, VT 05405-0059. Phone: 802-656-0827. E-mail: eseyler@zoo.uvm.edu.
- **Pennsylvania Farm Link:** Beginning Farmer Apprenticeship Program grants 144 hours per year of theoretical class instruction related to the selected trade and assigns apprentices of legal working age to a farm business employer in their chosen specialty. Participating farms must comply with the Fair Labor Standards Act. Housing may be provided to those who do not live within commuting distance of their placements. Contact: Marion Bowlan, Executive Director, 2708A North Colebrook Road, Manheim, PA 17545. Phone: 717-664-7077. E-mail: pafarmlink@redrose.net.
- **The Good Life Center:** A nonprofit organization dedicated to maintaining Helen and Scott Nearing's last hand-built home in Harborside, Maine, and sharing the philosophies of Helen and Scott Nearing. Offers visiting and residential fellowships, stewardships, and educational programs on homesteading and sustainable living. 372 Harborside Road, Harborside, ME 04642. Phone: 207-326-8211. Web site: <http://www.goodlife.com>.
- **Maysie's Farm Conservation Center:** Community-supported agriculture (CSA) program that produces organic food for 135 households on six acres. Maysie's Farm is a nonprofit educational conservation center that provides educational programs to CSA members and schools and offers an internship program that provides housing, a stipend, and organic food from the gardens. Contact: Sam Cantrell, Executive Director, 15 St. Andrew's Lane, Glenmoore, PA 19343. Phone: 610-458-8129. Web site: <http://www.maysiesfarm.org>.
- **Heron Pond Farm:** Contact Andre Cantelmo, 299 Main Avenue, South Hampton, NH 03728.
- **Land's Sake:** Initiated the nonprofit organization Green Power, a community farm project in Weston, Massachusetts, that offers a summer program to middle school students. Students grow fresh produce for homeless shelters and food pantries within the greater Boston area, receive a small stipend, and go on weekly educational field trips. Year-round environmental education workshops to the public are offered,

including maple sugaring and natural history field trips. P.O. Box 306, Weston, MA 02493. Phone: 781-893-1162.

- **The Delaware Valley Farm Study Center for Sustainable Living:** A nonprofit organization in eastern Pennsylvania that employs community children to work on a family-run vegetable farm and participate in weekly workshops during a summer program that integrates agriculture, art, and poetry. Each summer, the program focuses on a particular theme such as native plants or compassion for community, nature, and self. For more information, please write to Walt Schneiderwind and Jane Mayers at 6 Lodi Hill Road, Upper Black Eddy, PA 18972.

Agriculture Book Resources for Teaching

Bradley, Fern Marshall. *Rodale's All-New Encyclopedia of Organic Gardening.* 1992. Rodale Press, Emmaus, PA.

Bubel, Nancy. *The New Seed Starters Handbook.* 1988. Rodale Press, Emmaus, PA.

Carr, Anna. *Color Handbook of Garden Insects.* 1979. Rodale Press, Emmaus, PA.

Coleman, Eliot. *The Four Season Harvest.* Second Publishing, 1999. Chelsea Green, White River Junction, VT.

Coleman, Eliot. *The New Organic Grower: A Master's Manual of Tools and Techniques for the Home and Market Gardener.* 1989. Chelsea Green, White River Junction, VT.

Halpin, Anne. *Horticulture Gardener's Desk Reference.* 1996. Macmillan, New York.

Kiefer, Joseph and Kemple, Martin. *Digging Deeper, Integrating Youth Gardens into Schools and Communities.* 1998. Common Roots Press, Montpelier, VT.

Lee, Andrew W. *Backyard Market Gardening—The Entrepreneur's Guide to Selling What You Grow.* 1998. Good Earth Publications, Buena Vista, VA. Web site: <http://www.goodearthpub.com>.

Lerner, Carol. *My Backyard Garden.* 1998. Morrow Junior Books, New York.

Martin, Deborah L. and Gershuny, Grace (Eds.). *The Rodale Book of Composting—Easy Methods for Every Gardener.* 1992. Rodale Press, Emmaus, PA.

Mollison, Bill. *Introduction to Permaculture.* 1991. Tagari Publications, Tyalgum, Australia.

Moore, Barbara. *Growing with Gardening: A Twelve-Month Guide for Therapy, Recreation and Education.* 1989. University of North Carolina Press, Chapel Hill, NC.

National Gardening Association. *Grow Lab: Activities for Growing Minds* and *Grow Lab: A Complete Guide to Gardening in the Classroom.* 1990. Author, Burlington, VT.

Ocone, Lynn with Eve Pranis. *The National Gardening Association Guide to Kids' Gardening.* 1983. John Wiley and Sons, New York.

Parrella, Deborah. *Shelburne Farms Project Seasons—Hands-On Activities for Discovering the Wonders of the World.* 1995. Shelburne Farms, Shelburne, VT.

Richardson, Beth. *Gardening with Children.* 1998. Taunton Press, Newtown, CT.

Rogers, Marc. *Saving Seeds: The Gardener's Guide to Growing and Storing Vegetable and Flower Seeds.* 1990. Ecology Action, Willits, CA.

Salisbury, J. *The Green Classroom Program. A Teacher's Guide to a Garden-based Science Curriculum.* 1988. The New Alchemy Institute, East Falmouth, MA.

Smith, Miranda and Henderson, Elizabeth (Eds.). *The Real Dirt—Farmers Tell About Organic and Low-Input Practices in the Northeast.* 1994. Northeast Region Sustainable Agriculture Research and Education Program, Burlington, VT.

A Sample Agricultural Curriculum for High School Students

Weeks One and Two

History of agriculture—old and new world crops
Length of growing season for our area
Photosynthesis
Root structure, respiration, transpiration
Establish goals to donate produce to local food banks and sell at a local roadside stand
Activities: Garden planning and design—spring crops, germination, transplant, and harvest times of spring crops

Weeks Three and Four

Germination
Seed structure—i.e., embryo, cotyledon, endosperm
Monocot and dicot plants
Root structure—i.e., cortex, vascular rays, water transportation
Activities: Mix compost-based growing mix (peat moss, vibrant compost, vermiculite, lime, and powdered rock phosphate) for seedlings

Weeks Five and Six

Composting—nitrogen and carbon ratios
Compost versus soil absorption in glass cylinders
Activities: Plant kohlrabi, mustard, and chard seedlings

Note: All the information used to design these classes comes from resources cited in the appendixes.

Weeks Seven and Eight

Roles of three essential macronutrients: nitrogen, phosphate, and potassium

Soil composition: solids, liquids, and gases

Loamy soil requirements: sand, silt, and clay

Activities: Soil testing kit in the garden for pH, nitrogen, potassium, and phosphate; compare levels of compost versus soil; stratify layers of sand, silt, and clay in jars

Weeks Nine to Fifteen

Activities: Transplant seedlings to garden, mulch walkways, dig raised beds, direct sow seeds for fall crops (e.g., fall squashes), weed, water, harvest

Appendix D

A Sample Ecology Curriculum for High School Students

I taught this in three subsequent sessions: soil science, water quality, and forest ecology. Please review the resource guide in the appendixes as all of the following information can be found in these books.

Soil Science

Macronutrients (N-P-K: nitrogen, phosphorus, potassium) in soil and roles of each in plant development. Review micronutrients.

Review concept of nitrogen fixation.

Explain process of photosynthesis.

Define pH, review scale, ideal pH for plants.

Soil testing in garden for N-P-K using the LaMotte soil testing kit or No-Wait by Security Products Company (can be found on the Internet or through the National Gardening Association).

Soil composition: sand, silt, and clay. Can demonstrate stratification of layers by filling up a quart jar two-thirds full of water and add soil until the jar is full. The sand particles will settle on the bottom while silt and clay will take longer to settle. Use one teaspoon of a wetting agent, water softener, or liquid detergent to achieve the best stratification.

Study various soil samples from the forest and garden under a microscope. Compare particle size, texture, and weight. Record data.

Review aeration porosity (air and water exchange in soil particles).

Discuss soil erosion and nutrient cycle. Discuss the economic factors related to soil erosion.

Composting: Discuss the roles of nitrogen and carbon and what to add (i.e., fruit and vegetable scraps, leaves, twigs, etc).

Build a compost bin (read *Digging Deeper* by Joseph Kiefer and Martin Kemple).

Water Quality

Define and discuss the concept of watersheds.

Using Hach water testing kits (step-by-step instructions included), sample local creeks and test for pH, dissolved oxygen, and carbon dioxide. Other kits provide tests for nitrates and phosphates. Have students record data and formulate a report that includes all their collected data, a description of the location where testing took place and draw conclusions from some of the following questions:

- What does it mean if dissolved oxygen is present?
- What kind of stream life would we find here based on low or high levels of dissolved oxygen?
- What do you attribute to the level of dissolved oxygen? (i.e., think about climate, temperature, organic waste).
- Are these healthy creeks? Provide evidence for your answers.

Break students into groups and elect a spokesperson for each group. Hold a "town council" meeting and have elected spokespersons present their data. Manipulate the data (if necessary) to support evidence that creeks are not healthy. Come up with a plan to present to the town council that outlines solutions for improving water quality (i.e., petitioning community members, writing letters to local senators).

Call a local environmental council and find out if anyone is monitoring water quality in your area. This teaches students the concept of community, activism, and local culture, or simply, what is in their own backyards. Arrange a visit for this person to speak to your class or meet them on site. We met a woman who tested local creeks for nitrates and phosphates (our kit only had tests for pH, dissolved oxygen, and carbon dioxide). She was working to upgrade our local creeks and streams to an Exceptional Value (EV) status from High Quality (HQ). The EV rating offers the highest level of protection against possible pollution from developers (i.e., nitrates and phosphates from fertilizers that run into streams and creeks) and farms that use pesticides (also runs off into streams and creeks).

Students returned to class and wrote letters to a local senator asking him to support the EV rating. They were excited to receive an affirmative response that we read aloud in class.

Forest Ecology

Define stomata and guard cells. Examine leaf structure under microscopes. Explain the essential role of chloroplasts and chlorophyll.

A chromatography experiment will explain how chlorophyll masks the pigment in leaves. A simple classroom experiment requires acetone, test tubes, coffee filters, and various plant leaves. Detailed experiments can be found on the Internet by typing "chromatography" in any search engine.

Define the structure of the plant cell: nucleus, cytoplasm, vacuoles, and chloroplasts.

Hike through a nearby section of woods with a tree guide. Identify trees with opposite and alternate branching, define the difference between conifer and deciduous trees.

Explain the difference between simple and compound leaves, pinnately and palmately compound.

Discuss the inner layers of a tree (heartwood, sapwood, xylem, and phloem tissues).

Maple sugaring (read *The Amateur Sugar Maker* by Noel Perrin or *The Maple Sugar Book* by Helen and Scott Nearing). There are also many Web sites offering basic instructions on collecting and boiling sap over indoor stoves and outdoor fires, as well as building a makeshift evaporator, depending on your level of ambition!

Define root structure: epidermis, cortex, stele, and vascular rays.

Explain purposes of root structure: taproots, lateral/fibrous, and intermediate.

Define transpiration and the environmental factors that affect transpiration (humidity, temperature, and wind).

Collect leaves and store in a sealed bag for twenty-four hours to demonstrate transpiration.

Discuss interesting facts: a mature tree can release or transpire more than 200 gallons of water per day. A single corn plant can transpire two quarts or more of water in a day.

Appendix E

A Curriculum to Integrate Agriculture, Horticulture, and Environmental Concepts with Art

Art is an inherent part of nature. The fall forest is a splendor of foliage with maples, beeches, and oaks blanketing the forest floor with leaves of crimson, maize, and amber. A walk in the woods can provide inspiration and innumerable ideas for painting, sketching, and sculpture. Simple collages can be created from a variety of leaves. Found materials can be transformed into a sculpture and boulders provide the basis for a study on composition, detail, and light. Immersing oneself in nature provides a different perspective on art, one that is not often achieved in a traditional classroom setting. We traveled to four local areas of interest as described in further detail below.

Ringing Rocks is a local geological formation comprised of four acres of igneous boulders. When struck by a hammer, the rocks ring due to a high content of iron and aluminum. After sampling the various tones, students studied detail, composition, and light in charcoal studies.

A local stone sculptor collects a variety of stones and assembles them into a myriad of sculptures. A few pieces of limestone may be held together with epoxy or strategically balanced on top of each other to form an intriguing composition. Other pieces may be chiseled or carved. Steven kindly gave us a tour of the land around his house strewn with various sculptures. One student happily chiseled a piece of sandstone and others wandered around admiring Steven's work. During the next art class, we trekked through the woods and collected stones and twigs to create environmental sculptures. It was a successful venture with the exception of the epoxy, or "gorilla glue," that we used as it left several students scraping glue from their fingers for a day or two.

Hiking trails meander through the forest and wind around granite cliffs. Glimpsing down from the cliffs, the Tohickon Creek at High Rocks State Park winds it way through the canyon below. On a beautiful fall day, we hiked on foliage-covered trails down to the creek to capture the flow of water on paper using pastels.

The new Tinicum Aqueduct in Point Pleasant, Pennsylvania, provided the perfect study for perspective. Students chose locations such as the bridge and the creek to draw studies in colored pencil and pastels. Although perspective is a difficult concept for many students to grasp, it is essential for those who may want to pursue advanced drawing and painting classes.

Agriculture and Horticultural Art

Materials Needed

> charcoal pencils
> erasers
> drawing pencils
> oil pastels
> colored pencils
> paints/brushes/canvas boards

Session One

Review of essential concepts:

- Examples of impressionism (van Gogh, Seurat, Monet), realism (Wyeth), and abstract (Pollock, de Kooning, Kandinsky)
- Value and shading
- Seeing things as shapes and negative space
- Underpainting/underdrawing
- Composition and balance
- Color theory (review of primary colors, complementary colors, mixing various grays and greens)
- Perspective
- Cross hatching

Session Two

Seed Structure. Sketches in scrapbook using charcoal, colored pencils, or oil pastels. Brief overview of charcoal. Sketches to identify the internal structure of a seed: epicotyl, plumule, radicle, hypocotyl, and cotyledon. Sketch example of a monocot and dicot (i.e., corn and bean seeds).

Session Three

Flower Structure. Sketches in scrapbook using charcoal, colored pencils, or oil pastels. Sketches to identify the parts of a flower: stamen (anther, filament) and carpel (stigma, style, ovary).

Session Four

Leaf and Root Structure. Sketches in scrapbook using charcoal, colored pencils, or oil pastels. Sketches to identify the parts of a root: cortex, stele, epidermis, vascular rays. Sketches to identify leaf cells: xylem, phloem, stomata cells.

Session Five

Plant or Garden Studies. Using sketches from scrapbook and direct observation, students will produce two final paintings; one from this session and one in the subsequent session that will demonstrate an integration of skills learned in this course.

Session Six

Painted Flower and/or Vegetable Collage. Using sketches from scrapbook and direct observation, students will plan a painted collage comprised of flowers and/or vegetables. Color will be emphasized.

Notes

Preface

1. M. Norden, *Beyond Prozac* (New York: HarperCollins, 1995).
2. U. Timor, "Constructing a Rehabilitative Reality in Special Religious Wards in Israeli Prisons," *International Journal of Offender Therapy and Comparative Criminology* 42(4): 340-359.
3. Norden, *Beyond Prozac*.
4. H. Nearing and S. Nearing, *Living the Good Life* (New York: Schocken Books, 1970).

Chapter 1

1. American Psychiatric Association, *Diagnostic and Statistical Manual of Mental Disorders,* Fourth edition (Washington, DC: Author, 1994).
2. B.T. Zima, A.R. Perwien, T.R. Belin, and M. Widewski, "Children in Special Education Programs: ADHD Use of Services and Unmet Needs," *American Journal of Public Health* 88(6) (1998): 880-887.
3. D. Hellyer, A. Richardt, and J. Wenslaff, "School Intervention with Attention Deficit Hyperactivity Disorder," *School Social Work Journal* 21 (1997): 28-39.
4. Ibid.
5. M.K. Dulcan and S. Benson, "Summary of the Practice Parameters for the Assessment and Treatment of Children, Adolescents, and Adults with ADHD," *Journal of the American Academy of Child and Adolescent Psychiatry* 36(2) (1997): 1311-1317.
6. Hellyer, Richardt, and Wenslaff, "School Intervention with Attention Deficit Hyperactivity Disorder," p. 34.
7. J.J. Broderick-Cantwell, "Evaluation of ADHD Typology in Three Contrasting Samples: A Latent Class Approach," *Journal of the American Academy of Child and Adolescent Psychiatry* 38(1) (1999): 25-33.
8. Zima, Perwien, Belin, and Widewski, "Children in Special Education Programs."
9. T. Roszak, M. Gomes, and A. Kannes, *Ecopsychology: Restoring the Earth, Healing the Mind* (San Francisco, CA: The Sierra Club, 1995), p. 99.
10. D. Du Nann Winter, *Ecological Psychology: Healing the Split Between Planet and Self* (New York: HarperCollins, 1996).
11. K. Lewin, *Resolving Social Conflict and Field Theory in Social Science* (Washington, DC: American Psychological Association, 1997).
12. Du Nann Winter, *Ecological Psychology: Healing the Split Between Planet and Self.*

13. All Bible quotes are from *The Bible in Today's Version* (New York: The American Bible Society, 1976).

14. Du Nann Winter, *Ecological Psychology: Healing the Split Between Planet and Self.*

15. W. Berry, *The Unsettling of America: Culture and Agriculture* (San Francisco, CA: The Sierra Club, 1977).

16. A. Stoll, *The Omega-3 Connection* (New York: Simon and Schuster, 2001).

17. A.J. Zametkin and J. Rapoport, "Neurobiology of Attention Deficit Disorder with Hyperactivity: Where Have We Come in 50 Years?", *Journal of the American Academy of Child and Adolescent Psychiatry* 26 (1987): 676-686.

18. M.J. Norden, *Beyond Prozac* (New York: HarperCollins, 1995).

19. Ibid.

20. L.J. Mason, *Guide to Stress Reduction* (Berkeley, CA: Celestial Arts, 1985).

21. L.O. Bauer and V.M. Hesselbrock, "P300 Decrements in Teenagers with Conduct Problems: Implications for Substance Abuse Risk and Brain Development," *Biological Psychiatry* 46(2) (1999): 263-272.

22. E. Jocoy, J.E. Arruda, K. Estes, Y. Yagi, and K. Coburn, "Concurrent Visual Task Effects on Evoked and Emitted Auditory P300 in Adolescents," *International Journal of Psychophysiology* 30(3) (1998): 319-328.

23. A.P. Simopoulos and J. Robinson, *The Omega Diet* (New York: HarperCollins, 1999).

24. Bauer and Hesselbrock, "P300 Decrements in Teenagers with Conduct Problems."

25. Jocoy, Arruda, Estes, Yagi, and Coburn, "Concurrent Visual Task Effects on Evoked and Emitted Auditory P300 in Adolescents."

26. Ibid.

27. B.G. Winsberg, "Electrophysiological Indices of Information Processing in Methylphenidate Responders," *Biological Psychiatry* 42(6) (1997): 434-445.

28. M. Matsuura, Y. Okubo, M. Toru, T. Kojima, Y. He, Y. Hou, Y. Shen, and C.K. Lee, "A Cross-National EEG Study of Children with Emotional and Behavioral Problems: A WHO Collaborative Study in the Western Pacific Region," *Biological Psychiatry* 34(1/2) (1993): 59-65.

29. Bauer and Hesselbrock, "P300 Decrements in Teenagers with Conduct Problems."

30. S. Kuperman, B. Johnson, S. Arndt, S. Lindgren, and M. Wolraich, "Quantitative EEG Differences in a Nonclinical Sample of Children with ADHD and Undifferentiated ADD," *Journal of the American Academy of Child and Adolescent Psychiatry* 35(8) (1996): 1009-1117.

31. Matsuura, Okubo, Toru, Kojima, He, Hou, Shen, and Lee, "A Cross-National EEG Study of Children with Emotional and Behavioral Problems."

32. Mason, *Guide to Stress Reduction.*

33. J. Bennington and J. Polich, "Comparison of P300 from Passive and Active Tasks for Auditory and Visual Stimuli," *International Journal of Psychophysiology* 34(2) (1999): 171-177.

34. Jocoy, Arruda, Estes, Yagi, and Coburn, "Concurrent Visual Task Effects on Evoked and Emitted Auditory P300 in Adolescents."

35. Ibid.

36. R. Kilpelainen, L. Luoma, E. Herrgard, H. Ypparila, J. Partanen, and J. Karhu, "Persistent Frontal P300 Brain Potential Suggests Abnormal Processing of Auditory Information in Distractible Children," *Neuroreport* 10(16) (1999): 3405-3410.

37. Bauer and Hesselbrock, "P300 Decrements in Teenagers with Conduct Problems."

38. Simopoulos and Robinson, *The Omega Diet.*

39. P.J. Murthy, V. Naga, B.N. Gangadhar, N. Janakiramaiah, and D.K. Subbakrishna, "Normalization of P300 Amplitude Following Treatment in Dysthymia," *Biological Psychiatry* 42(8) (1997): 740-743.

40. A.J. Zametkin and M. Ernst, "Problems in the Management of Attention Deficit Hyperactivity Disorder," *New England Journal of Medicine* 340(1) (1999): 40-46.

41. J. Elia, P.J. Ambrosini, and J.L. Rapoport, "Treatment of Attention Deficit Hyperactivity Disorder," *New England Journal of Medicine* 340(10) (1999): 780-788, p. 780.

42. C. Barr, "Genetics of Childhood Disorders: XXII. ADHD, Part 6: The Dopamine D4 Receptor Gene," *Journal of the American Academy of Child & Adolescent Psychiatry* 40(1) (2001): 118-121.

43. Ibid.

44. D. Amen, *Change Your Brain, Change Your Life* (New York: Three Rivers Press, 1998).

45. Ibid.

46. Ibid.

47. Ibid.

48. Norden, *Beyond Prozac.*

49. G.J. DuPaul, T.L. Eckert, and K.E. McGoey, "Interventions for Students With ADHD: One Size Does Not Fit All," *School Psychology Review* 26(3) (1997): 369-381.

50. C. Carlson, W. Pelham, R. Milich, and J. Dixon, "Single and Combined Effects of Methylphenidate and Behavior Therapy on the Classroom Performance of Children with Attention Deficit Hyperactivity Disorder," *Journal of Abnormal Child Psychology* 20(2) (1992): 213-232.

51. C. Hannaford, *Smart Moves* (Arlington, VA: Great Ocean Publishers, 1995).

52. K. Zernike and M. Petersen, "Schools' Backing of Behavior Drugs Comes Under Fire," *The New York Times* August 19 (2001): A1+.

53. Ibid.

54. Ibid.

55. J.O. Prochaska and C.C. DiClemente, "In Search of How People Change: Applications to Addictive Behaviors," *American Psychologist* 47(9) (1992): 1102-1114.

56. D.H. Hepworth, R.H. Rooney, and J.A. Larsen, *Direct Social Work Practice: Theory and Skills,* Third Edition (Belmont, CA: Brooks/Cole Publishing, 1997).

57. D. Saleeby, *The Strengths Perspective in Social Work Practice,* Second Edition (New York: Longman, 1997).

Chapter 2

1. Decisional balances are a concept developed by G.A. Marlatt. For more information, see F. Rotgers, *Innovations in Clinical Practice: A Source Book* (Volume 16) (Sarasota, FL: Professional Resource Exchange, 1982).

2. W. R. Miller, "Why Do People Change Addictive Behavior? The 1996 H. David Archibald Lecture," *Addiction* 93(2) (1998): 163-172. Developing discrepancy is a therapeutic process that enhances salient awareness of the cons of current behavior and the pros of change. If people become engaged in positive, interesting, and intellectually stimulating activities where persistent drug and alchohol use hinders their progress, a consciousness of the disadvantages of continued use may suddenly become apparent. Other similar effective techniques include a three-column record of a situation, with thoughts and feelings during a craving or urge to use a substance that one is attempting to quit. By examining the situation in retrospect during a session, a client is able to recognize the thoughts and feelings, understand the situation, and think of alternative ways to cope in a future situation. Another strategy is to devise an emergency plan to be used during overwhelming feelings of emotions, situations, or intense cravings. This includes a list of people to contact as well as a list of alternative activities to pursue. For example, a brainstorming session during one hour elicited a creative list of one client's favorite activities, which included researching nutrition, taking a computer course, and playing a musical instrument. Furthermore, I requested that this particular client spend thirty to sixty minutes daily engaged in such an activity to raise conscious awareness that pleasurable activities in lieu of drinking do not have the same negative consequences.

3. Civil Immunity Act, Chapter 270, Senate No. 3063.

4. B.S. McCann, T.L. Simpson, R. Ries, and P. Roy-Byrne, "Reliability and Validity of Screening Instruments for Drug and Alcohol Abuse Adults Seeking Evaluation for Attention Deficit Hyperactivity Disorder," *American Journal on Addictions* 9(1) (2000): 1-9.

5. F.R. Levin and S.M. Evans, "Diagnostic and Treatment Issues in Comorbid Substance Abuse and Adult Attention Deficit Hyperactivity Disorder," *Psychiatric Annals* 31(5) (2001): 303-312.

6. J. Biederman, T.E. Wilens, E. Mick, S.V. Faraone, and T. Spencer, "Does Attention Deficit Hyperactivity Disorder Impact the Developmental Course of Drug and Alcohol Abuse and Dependence?" *Biological Psychiatry* 44(4) (1998): 269-273.

7. J. Elia, P.J. Ambrosini, and J.L. Rapoport, "Treatment of Attention Deficit Hyperactivity Disorder," *New England Journal of Medicine* 340(10) (1999): 780-788.

8. M.T. Lynskey and W. Hall, "Attention Deficit Hyperactivity Disorder and Substance Use Disorder: Is There a Causal Link?" *Addiction* 96(6) (2001): 815-822.

9. Levin and Evans, "Diagnostic and Treatment Issues in Comorbid Substance Abuse and Adult Attention Deficit Hyperactivity Disorder."

10. Ibid.

11. P. Tucker, "Attention Deficit Hyperactivity Disorder in the Drug and Alcohol Clinic," *Drug and Alcohol Review* 18(3) (1999): 337-344.

12. Lynskey and Hall, "Attention Deficit Hyperactivity Disorder and Substance Use Disorder: Is There a Causal Link?"

13. Ibid.

14. Tucker, "Attention Deficit Hyperactivity Disorder in the Drug and Alcohol Clinic."

15. Biederman, Wilens, Mick, Faraone, and Spencer, "Does Attention Deficit Hyperactivity Disorder Impact the Developmental Course of Drug and Alcohol Abuse and Dependence?"

16. Committee on Child Health Financing and Committee on Substance Abuse, "Improving Substance Abuse Prevention, Assessment and Treatment Financing for Children and Adolescents," *Pediatrics* 108(4) (2001): 1025-1029.

17. B.S. McCann, T.L. Simpson, R. Ries, and P. Roy-Byrne, "Reliability and Validity of Screening Instruments for Drug and Alcohol Abuse Adults Seeking Evaluation for Attention Deficit Hyperactivity Disorder," *American Journal on Addictions* 9(1) (2000): 1-9.

18. Lynskey and Hall, "Attention Deficit Hyperactivity Disorder and Substance Use Disorder: Is There a Causal Link?"

19. Levin and Evans, "Diagnostic and Treatment Issues in Comorbid Substance Abuse and Adult Attention Deficit Hyperactivity Disorder."

20. Ibid, p. 309.

21. Ibid.

22. Ibid.

23. S. Stukin, "Freedom from Addiction," *Yoga Journal* June (2002): 47-55.

24. Miller, "Why Do People Change Addictive Behavior?"

25. J.O. Prochaska and C.C. DiClemente, "In Search of How People Change: Applications to Addictive Behaviors," *American Psychologist* 47(9) (1992): 1102-1114.

26. See Rotgers, *Innovations in Clinical Practice,* for a more detailed explanation of harm reduction.

27. Miller, "Why Do People Change Addictive Behavior?"

28. Rotgers, *Innovations in Clinical Practice.*

Chapter 3

1. H.R. Samuel, "Impediments to Implementing Environmental Education," *Journal of Environmental Education* 25(1) (1993): 26-29, p. 27.

2. P. Eagles and M. Richardson, "The Status of Environmental Education at Field Centers of Ontario Schools," *Journal of Environmental Education* 23(4) (1992): 9-14, p. 10.

3. D.W. Orr, *Ecological Literacy: Education and the Transition to a Postmodern World.*

4. Eagles and Richardson, "The Status of Environmental Education at Field Centers of Ontario Schools."

5. T. Roszak, M. Gomes, and A. Kannes, *Ecopsychology: Restoring the Earth, Healing the Mind* (San Francisco, CA: The Sierra Club, 1995).

6. H.D. Thoreau, *Walden* (Ware, Hertfordshire: Wordsworth Editions Limited, 1995), p. 35.

7. See Appendix A for contact information.

8. Roszak, Gomes, and Kannes, *Ecopsychology.*

9. J. Jobb, *The Complete Book of Community Gardening* (New York: Morrow, 1979).

10. National Gardening Association, "Self-Esteem, Social Skills, Behavior," *Growing Ideas* 11(1) (2000): 1-12.

11. Ibid.

12. P. Fry and E. Yellin, "The Therapeutic Garden," *Teaching Tolerance* (1999): 46-51.

13. B. Donahue, *Reclaiming the Commons: Community Farms and Forests in a New England Town* (New Haven, CT: Yale University Press, 1999), p. 95.

14. Ibid., p. 96.

15. N.J. Smith-Sebasto and T.L. Smith, "Environmental Education in Illinois and Wisconsin: A Tale of Two States," *Journal of Environmental Education* 28(4) (1997): 26-36.

16. M. Roy, R. Petty, and R. Durgin, "Traveling Boxes: A New Tool for Environmental Education," *Journal of Environmental Education* 28(4) (1997): 9-17.

17. D. Hellyer, A. Richardt, and J. Wenslaff, "School Intervention with Attention Deficit Hyperactivity Disorder," *School Social Work Journal* 21 (1997): 28-39.

18. C. Hannaford, *Smart Moves* (Arlington, VA: Great Ocean Publishers, 1995).

19. Ibid.

20. Ibid.

21. L. Sewall, *Sight and Sensibility: The Ecopsychology of Perception* (New York: Tarcher/Putnam Books, 1999), p. 280.

22. D. Orr, "What Is Education For?" *Annals of Earth* VIII(2) (1990).

23. F. Capra, *The Web of Life* (New York: Anchor Books, 1996).

24. J. Gambro and H. Switzy, "A National Survey of High School Students' Environmental Knowledge," *Journal of Environmental Education* 27(3) (1996): 28-33.

25. Ibid.

26. J. Lane, R. Wilke, R. Champeau, and D. Sivek, "Environmental Education in Wisconsin: A Teacher Survey," *Journal of Environmental Education* 25(4) (1994): 9-17.

27. Smith-Sebasto and Smith, "Environmental Education in Illinois and Wisconsin."

28. Eagles and Richardson, "The Status of Environmental Education at Field Centers of Ontario Schools."

29. Orr, *Ecological Literacy.*

30. Ibid.

31. W. Berry, *The Unsettling of America: Culture and Agriculture* (San Francisco, CA: The Sierra Club, 1977), p. 157.

32. K. Lewin, *Resolving Social Conflicts and Field Theory in Social Science* (Washington, DC: American Psychological Association, 1997).

33. D. Kunz-Shuman and S. Ham, "Toward a Theory of Commitment to Environmental Education Teaching," *Journal of Environmental Education* 28(2) (1997): 25-32.

34. Ibid.

35. Orr, *Ecological Literacy.*

36. B.F. Skinner, *Beyond Freedom and Dignity* (New York: Bantam Books, 1971), p. 201.

37. Ibid.

38. W. Berry, *The Gift of Good Land* (Canada: HarperCollinsCanadaLtd, 1981), pp. 280-281.

Chapter 4

1. M.J. Norden, *Beyond Prozac* (New York: HarperCollins, 1995).

2. W. Berry, *The Unsettling of America: Culture and Agriculture* (San Francisco, CA: The Sierra Club, 1977), p. 138.

3. N. Cusano, "Learning to Grow," *The Boston Sunday Globe* August 27 (2000): E2.

4. E. Henderson, *Sharing the Harvest* (White River Junction, VT: Chelsea Green Publishing, 1999).

5. N. Bloch, "In Harm's Way," *Earthwatch* May/June (1998): 8-9.

6. A. Cichoke, *Enzymes and Enzyme Therapy* (Chicago, IL: Keats Publishing, 1994).

7. Ibid.

8. D. Du Nann Winter, *Ecological Psychology: Healing the Split Between Planet and Self* (New York: HarperCollins, 1996).

9. Henderson, *Sharing the Harvest*.

10. B. Jensen, *Foods That Heal* (New York: Avery Publishing Group, 1993).

11. F. Diez-Gonzalez, T. Callaway, M. Kizoulis, and J. Russell, "Grain Feeding and the Dissemination of Acid-Resistant Escherichia Coli from Cattle," *Science* 281(5383) (1998): 1666-1668.

12. Henderson, *Sharing the Harvest*.

13. Berry, *The Unsettling of America*.

14. D. Orr, *Earth in Mind* (Washington, DC: Island Press, 1994).

15. A. Stoll, *The Omega-3 Connection* (New York: Simon and Schuster, 2001).

16. A.P. Simopoulos and J. Robinson, *The Omega Diet* (New York: HarperCollins 1999).

17. Ibid.

18. R. Gibson, "Long Chain Polyunsaturated Fatty Acids and Infant Development," *The Lancet* 354(9194) (1999): 1919-1920.

19. L.J. Stevens, S.S. Zentall, M.L. Abate, T. Kuczek, and J.R. Burgess, "Omega-3 Fatty Acid Status in Boys with Behavior, Learning and Health Problems," *Physiology and Behavior* 59 (1996): 915-920.

20. Stoll, *The Omega-3 Connection*.

21. Ibid.

22. Gibson, "Long Chain Polyunsaturated Fatty Acids and Infant Development."

23. Ibid.

24. Simopoulos and Robinson, *The Omega Diet*.

25. Ibid.

26. Stoll, *The Omega-3 Connection*.

27. Simopoulos and Robinson, *The Omega Diet*.

28. Jensen, *Foods That Heal*.

29. M. Coleman, G. Steinberg, J. Tippett, H.N. Bhagavan, D.B. Coursin, M. Gross, C. Lewis, and L. DeVeau, "A Preliminary Study of the Effect of Pyridoxine Administration in a Subgroup of Hyperkinetic Children: A Double-Blind Crossover Comparison with Methylphenidate," *Biological Psychiatry* 14(5) (1979): 741-751.

30. M.A. Block, "Attention on Kids," *Energy Times* 10(9) (2000): 43-47.

31. H.E. Thelander, J.K. Phelps, and K. Walton, "Learning Disabilities Associated with Lesser Brain Damage," *Journal of Pediatrics* 53 (1958): 405-409.

32. J. Gallo, "Enzymes," *Energy Times* 9(10) (1999): 25-30.

33. A. Demas, *Food is Elementary: A Hands-On Curriculum for Young Students* (New York: Food Studies Institute, 1999). Curriculum integrating academic disciplines with food, nutrition, culture, and the arts. This study is the Cornell University doctoral thesis of Dr. Antonia Demas.

34. Orr, *Earth in Mind,* p. 120.

Chapter 5

1. C.S. Lewis, *Mere Christianity* (New York: Macmillan Publishing, 1943), p. 75.

2. A. Maslow, *Religions, Values and Peak Experiences* (Dallas, PA: Kappa Delta Pi, 1964).

3. Lewis, *Mere Christianity,* p. 136.

4. C.R. Swenson, "Clinical Practice and the Decline of Community," *Journal of Teaching in Social Work* 10(1/2) (1994): 195-211.

5. P. Cushman, "Why the Self Is Empty," *American Psychologist* 45(5) (1990): 599-611.

6. M. Burke, H. Hackney, P. Hudson, and J. Miranti, "Spirituality, Religion and CACREP Curriculum Standards," *Journal of Counseling and Development* 77(3) (1999): 251-257.

7. D.N. Elkins, "Spirituality: It's What's Missing in Mental Health," *Psychology Today* 32(5) (1999): 45-48.

8. T. Cascio, "Incorporating Spirituality into Social Work Practice: A Review of What to Do," *Families in Society: The Journal of Contemporary Human Services* 79 (1998): 523-531.

9. Elkins, "Spirituality: It's What's Missing in Mental Health," p. 47.

10. Lewis, *Mere Christianity,* p. 52.

11. Maslow, *Religions, Values and Peak Experiences,* p. 75.

12. Ibid.

13. J. Ziegler, "Spirituality Returns to the Fold in Medical Practice," *Journal of National Cancer Institute* 90 (1998): 1255-1257.

14. R. Sloan, E. Bagiella, and T. Powell, "Religion, Spirituality and Medicine," *The Lancet* 353 (1999): 664-667.

15. Elkins, "Spirituality: It's What's Missing in Mental Health."

16. Burke, Hackney, Hudson, and Miranti, "Spirituality, Religion and CACREP Curriculum Standards."

17. Sloan, Bagiella, and Powell, "Religion, Spirituality and Medicine."

18. U. Timor, "Constructing a Rehabilitative Reality in Special Religious Wards in Israeli Prisons," *International Journal of Offender Therapy and Comparative Criminology* 42(4) (1998): 340-359.

19. Timor, "Constructing a Rehabilitative Reality in Special Religious Wards in Israeli Prisons."

20. L. White, Jr., "The Historical Roots of Our Ecological Crisis," *Science* 155(3767) (1967): 1203-1207.

21. D.B. Fink, "Judaism and Ecology: A Theology of Creation," *Earth Ethics* 10(1) (1998): 6-7.

22. D.T. Hessel, "Christianity and Ecology: Wholeness, Respect, Justice, Sustainability," *Earth Ethics* 10(1) (1998): 8-9.

23. M. Marangudakis, "Ecology As a Pseudo-Religion?" *Telos* 112 (1998): 107-125.

24. J. Moehlmann, "The Religious Community and the Environment," *Bioscience* 42(8) (1992): 627.

25. B. Barcott, "For God So Loved the World," *The Utne Reader* August (2001): 50-56.

26. Ibid.

Chapter 6

1. W. Berry, *The Unsettling of America: Culture and Agriculture* (San Francisco, CA: The Sierra Club, 1977), p. 138.

2. M. Burke, H. Hackney, P. Hudson, and J. Miranti, "Spirituality, Religion and CACREP Curriculum Standards," *Journal of Counseling and Development* 77(3) (1999): 251-257.

3. T. Berry, *Dream of the Earth* (San Franciso, CA: Sierra Club Books, 1990), p. 37.

4. T. Roszak, M. Gomes, and A. Kannes, *Ecopsychology: Restoring the Earth, Healing the Mind* (San Francisco, CA: The Sierra Club, 1995).

5. D. Ehrenfeld, *Beginning Again: People and Nature in the New Millennium* (New York: Oxford University Press, 1995), p. 20.

6. Roszak, Gomes, and Kannes, *Ecopsychology,* p. 226.

7. W. Myers, P. Burton, P. Sanders, K. Donat, J. Cheney, T. Fitzpatrick, and L. Monaco, "Project Back-on-Track at 1 Year: A Delinquency Treatment Program for Early Career Juvenile Offenders," *Journal of the American Academy of Child and Adolescent Psychiatry* 39(9) (2000): 1127-1134.

8. The Center for Rural Pennsylvania, "Pennsylvania's Rural Homeless Reality," *Rural Perspectives* 9(6) (2000): 1-8.

9. Report published by Bowers Publishing, Inc., that is based on information from interviews with county administrators in July 2000 and the USDA's 1997 Census of Agriculture.

10. J. McCommons, "Humus and Humility," *Organic Gardening* 48(5) (2001): 26-30.

11. B. Barnes, "Sharing in the Harvest," *Philadelphia Inquirer* August 1 (1999): CC1+.

12. B. Barnes, "To Save His Farm, He Needs the Community," *Philadelphia Inquirer* May 5 (1999): B1+.

Chapter 7

1. L.J. Mason, *Guide to Stress Reduction* (Berkeley, CA: Celestial Arts, 1985).

2. D. Du Nann Winter, *Ecological Psychology: Healing the Split Between Planet and Self* (New York: HarperCollins, 1996).

3. Ibid.

4. C. Hannaford, *Smart Moves* (Arlington, VA: Great Ocean Publishers, 1995).

5. M. Brinkerhoff and J. Jacob, "Mindfulness and Quasi-Religious Meaning Systems: An Empirical Exploration Within the Context of Ecological Sustainability and Deep Ecology," *Journal for the Scientific Study of Religion* 38(4) (1999): 524-543.

6. L. Sewall, *Sight and Sensibility: The Ecopsychology of Perception* (New York: Tarcher/Putnam Books, 1999).

7. T. Cleary, *The Five Houses of Zen* (Boston, MA: Shambhala, 1997).

8. Ibid.

9. M. Munitz, *The Ways of Philosophy* (New York: Macmillan Publishing, 1979), p. 325.

10. Ibid.

11. T. Northcut, "Soul on the Couch: Spirituality, Religion and Morality in Contemporary Psychoanalysis," *Clinical Social Work Journal* 27(2) (1999): 217-220.

12. D.N. Elkins, "Spirituality: It's What's Missing in Mental Health," *Psychology Today* 32(5) (1999): 45-48.

13. T. Szasz, *The Myth of Mental Illness: Foundations of a Theory of Personal Conduct* (New York: HarperCollins, 1984).

14. Sewall, *Sight and Sensibility.*

15. T. Roszak, M. Gomes, and A. Kannes, *Ecopsychology: Restoring the Earth, Healing the Mind* (San Francisco, CA: The Sierra Club, 1995).

16. C. Collins, "Yoga: Intuition, Preventive Medicine, and Treatment," *Journal of Obstetric, Gynecologic, and Neonatal Nursing* 27(5): 563-568.

17. R. Schaeffer, *Yoga for Your Spiritual Muscles* (Wheaton, IL: Quest Books, 1998).

18. J. Gold, "Plato in the Light of Yoga," *Philosophy East and West* 46(1) (1996): 17-33.

19. B. Edwards, *Drawing on the Artist Within* (New York: Simon & Schuster, 1986).

20. Collins, "Yoga: Intuition, Preventive Medicine, and Treatment."

21. Ibid.

22. Schaeffer, *Yoga for Your Spiritual Muscles.*

23. Collins, "Yoga: Intuition, Preventive Medicine, and Treatment."

24. Mason, *Guide to Stress Reduction.*

25. P. Murthy, B. Gangadhar, N. Jahakiramaiah, and D. Subbakrishna, "Normalization of P300 Amplitude Following Treatment in Dysthymia," *Biological Psychiatry* 42(8) (1997): 740-743.

26. Roszak, Gomes, and Kannes, *Ecopsychology.*

Chapter 8

1. P. Keller, *A Shepherd Looks at Psalm 23* (Grand Rapids, MI: Zondervan Publishing House, 1970), p. 20.

2. Ibid, p. 21.

Index

Printed and bound by CPI Group (UK) Ltd, Croydon, CR0 4YY

23/10/2024

01778117-0001